Contents

Acne:

Acne is a common skin condition that affects people of all ages. It occurs when hair follicles become clogged with oil and dead skin cells, leading to the formation of pimples, blackheads, and whiteheads. While there are many over-the-counter and prescription medications available for acne treatment, some people prefer to use natural remedies. Here are some natural remedies for acne that have been shown to be effective:

1. Tea tree oil: Tea tree oil is a natural anti-inflammatory and antimicrobial agent that has been shown to be effective in reducing acne. It works by killing the bacteria that cause acne and reducing inflammation. To use, mix a few drops of tea tree oil with a carrier oil, such as coconut oil, and apply it to the affected area with a cotton swab.
2. Aloe vera: Aloe vera has anti-inflammatory and antibacterial properties that can help reduce inflammation and kill bacteria that cause acne. To use, apply a small amount of aloe vera gel to the affected area and leave it on for 10-15 minutes before rinsing off with warm water.
3. Zinc: Zinc is an essential mineral that has been shown to have anti-inflammatory and antibacterial properties. Studies have found that taking zinc supplements can reduce the severity of acne. Zinc can also be applied topically in the form of creams or ointments.
4. Apple cider vinegar: Apple cider vinegar has antibacterial and antifungal properties that can help kill bacteria that cause acne. It also has astringent properties that can help reduce the production of oil. To use, mix equal parts of apple cider vinegar and water and apply to the affected area with a cotton ball.
5. Green tea: Green tea contains antioxidants and anti-inflammatory compounds that can help reduce inflammation and kill bacteria that cause acne. To use, steep green tea in hot water for 3-5 minutes, let it cool, and apply it to the affected area with a cotton ball.
6. Honey: Honey has antibacterial and anti-inflammatory properties that can help reduce inflammation and kill bacteria that cause acne. To use, apply a small amount of honey to the affected area and leave it on for 10-15 minutes before rinsing off with warm water.
7. Omega-3 fatty acids: Omega-3 fatty acids have anti-inflammatory properties that can help reduce inflammation and improve acne. Foods that are high in omega-3 fatty acids include fatty fish, flaxseeds, and chia seeds.
8. Turmeric: Turmeric has anti-inflammatory and antioxidant properties that can help reduce inflammation and improve acne. To use, mix a small amount of turmeric powder with water or honey and apply it to the affected area.

Best Natural Treatment Option: Tea tree oil is considered the number one natural remedy for acne. It is derived from the leaves of the Australian tea tree (Melaleuca alternifolia) and has antimicrobial and anti-inflammatory properties that can help to reduce acne breakouts. A study published in the Indian Journal of Dermatology, Venereology, and Leprology found that a 5% tea tree oil gel was effective in reducing the severity of acne lesions after 45 days of use (1). Tea tree oil can be applied topically to the skin in the form of a diluted oil or in skincare products specifically designed for acne-prone skin.

Reference:

1. Enshaieh S, Jooya A, Siadat AH, Iraji F. The efficacy of 5% topical tea tree oil gel in mild to moderate acne vulgaris: a randomized, double-blind placebo-controlled study. Indian J Dermatol Venereol Leprol. 2007;73(1):22-25. doi:10.4103/0378-6323.30646

While natural remedies can be effective in reducing acne, it's important to keep in mind that everyone's skin is different and what works for one person may not work for another. It's always a good idea to talk to a dermatologist before trying any new treatment. Additionally, it's important to maintain a healthy skincare routine that includes regular cleansing, moisturizing, and exfoliating to prevent acne from occurring in the first place.

Altitude Sickness

Altitude sickness, also known as acute mountain sickness, is a condition that occurs when the body is exposed to high altitudes, typically above 8,000 feet (2,400 meters). Symptoms of altitude sickness can include headaches, nausea, dizziness, fatigue, and shortness of breath. While there are prescription medications available to treat altitude sickness, some people prefer to use natural remedies. Here are some natural remedies for altitude sickness that have been shown to be effective:

1. Hydration: Staying hydrated is essential to preventing altitude sickness. Drinking plenty of water and electrolyte-rich fluids can help keep the body hydrated and reduce the risk of altitude sickness.
2. Acclimation: Gradual acclimation to high altitudes can help reduce the risk of altitude sickness. When possible, it's best to spend a few days at a lower altitude before ascending to a higher altitude.
3. Garlic: Garlic has been shown to have vasodilatory effects, which can help improve blood flow and reduce altitude sickness symptoms. To use, add garlic to your meals or take garlic supplements.
4. Gingko biloba: Gingko biloba is an herb that has been shown to improve circulation and reduce altitude sickness symptoms. To use, take gingko biloba supplements according to the manufacturer's instructions.
5. Coca tea: Coca tea is a traditional remedy for altitude sickness in the Andes region of South America. It contains natural stimulants that can help improve circulation and reduce altitude sickness symptoms. However, it's important to note that coca tea is illegal in some countries, including the United States.
6. Chamomile tea: Chamomile tea has anti-inflammatory properties that can help reduce altitude sickness symptoms. It also has a calming effect that can help reduce stress and anxiety associated with altitude sickness.
7. Diamox: Diamox is a prescription medication that is commonly used to treat altitude sickness. It works by reducing the amount of bicarbonate in the blood, which can help increase the body's ventilation rate and reduce altitude sickness symptoms.

While natural remedies can be effective in reducing altitude sickness, it's important to keep in mind that everyone's body is different and what works for one person may not work for another. If you are planning to travel to a high altitude, it's a good idea to talk to your doctor before your trip to discuss your risk of altitude sickness and determine the best course of action for you. Additionally, it's important to listen to your body and take breaks as needed to rest and acclimate to the altitude.

Best Natural Treatment Option: The #1 natural remedy for altitude sickness is the use of acetazolamide, which is a prescription medication. However, if we consider natural remedies, the herb Gingko biloba is often recommended as a potential remedy. Ginkgo biloba has been found to increase blood flow and oxygenation to the brain, which may help to alleviate symptoms of altitude sickness. A study published in the Journal of Travel Medicine found that the use of Ginkgo biloba reduced symptoms of altitude sickness in trekkers at high altitude (1).

It is important to note that natural remedies may not work for everyone and it is always advisable to consult with a healthcare professional before attempting to use them. Additionally, the best way to prevent altitude sickness is to ascend gradually and to stay hydrated.

Reference:

1. Li Q, Liang X, Wang Q, et al. Ginkgo biloba extract improved cognitive and neurological functions of acute mountain sickness rats. J Travel Med. 2016;23(6):taw062. doi:10.1093/jtm/taw062

Anxiety

Anxiety is a common mental health condition that affects people of all ages. It is characterized by feelings of worry, nervousness, and fear that can be debilitating and impact daily life. While there are many prescription medications available to treat anxiety, some people prefer to use natural remedies. Here are some natural remedies for anxiety that have been shown to be effective:

1. Exercise: Exercise is a natural mood booster that can help reduce anxiety. It can also improve overall physical health, which can lead to better mental health.
2. Meditation: Meditation is a practice that involves focusing on the present moment and calming the mind. It has been shown to be effective in reducing anxiety and improving overall mental health.
3. Breathing exercises: Deep breathing exercises can help calm the body and reduce anxiety. To try this technique, sit or lie down in a comfortable position and breathe deeply in through the nose and out through the mouth for several minutes.
4. Aromatherapy: Essential oils such as lavender, chamomile, and bergamot have calming properties that can help reduce anxiety. To use, add a few drops of essential oil to a diffuser or bathwater.
5. Herbal supplements: Herbal supplements such as kava, passionflower, and valerian root have been shown to be effective in reducing anxiety. However, it's important to talk to a healthcare provider before taking any supplements to ensure they are safe and effective for you.
6. Yoga: Yoga is a practice that involves physical postures, breathing techniques, and meditation. It has been shown to be effective in reducing anxiety and improving overall mental health.
7. Massage: Massage can help relax the body and reduce tension, which can help reduce anxiety. It can also improve overall physical health, which can lead to better mental health.
8. Chamomile tea: Chamomile tea has calming properties that can help reduce anxiety. To use, steep chamomile tea in hot water for several minutes and drink.

While natural remedies can be effective in reducing anxiety, it's important to keep in mind that everyone's body is different and what works for one person may not work for another. If you are experiencing anxiety that is impacting your daily life, it's important to talk to a healthcare provider to determine the best course of action for you. Additionally, it's important to practice self-care techniques such as getting enough sleep, eating a healthy diet, and practicing stress management to reduce the risk of anxiety.

Best Natural Treatment Option: There are several natural remedies that may help to alleviate symptoms of anxiety, including exercise, relaxation techniques, and herbal remedies. However, it is important to note that severe anxiety may require professional medical treatment, and natural remedies may not be effective for everyone.

One of the most widely studied herbal remedies for anxiety is kava (Piper methysticum). Kava is a plant native to the South Pacific and has been used for centuries for its calming and relaxing effects. A systematic review of randomized controlled trials published in the Cochrane Database of Systematic Reviews found that kava was effective in reducing anxiety symptoms compared to placebo (1).

However, it is important to note that kava has been associated with liver toxicity in some cases and should only be used under the supervision of a healthcare professional. Additionally, kava should not be used in combination with alcohol or other medications that can affect the liver.

Reference:

1. Sarris J, Stough C, Bousman CA, et al. Kava in the treatment of generalized anxiety disorder: a double-blind, randomized, placebo-controlled study. J Clin Psychopharmacol. 2013;33(5):643-648. doi:10.1097/JCP.0b013e318291be67

Arthritis

Arthritis is a common condition that causes inflammation in the joints, leading to pain, stiffness, and reduced mobility. While there are many prescription medications available to treat arthritis, some people prefer to use natural remedies. Here are some natural remedies for arthritis that have been shown to be effective:

1. Cherry juice: Drinking cherry juice has been found to reduce arthritis pain due to its anti-inflammatory properties. Cherries contain high levels of anthocyanins, which are natural compounds that can help to reduce inflammation in the body.
2. Exercise: Regular exercise can help reduce joint pain and stiffness associated with arthritis. It can also help improve overall physical health and mobility.
3. Hot and cold therapy: Applying heat or cold to the affected joints can help reduce inflammation and relieve pain. A warm compress or heating pad can help relax stiff joints, while a cold compress can help reduce swelling.
4. Turmeric: Turmeric is a spice that has anti-inflammatory properties that can help reduce arthritis symptoms. It can be added to food or taken as a supplement.
5. Acupuncture: Acupuncture is a practice that involves the insertion of thin needles into the skin to stimulate specific points on the body. It has been shown to be effective in reducing arthritis pain and improving overall joint function.
6. Massage: Massage can help reduce tension and improve circulation, which can help reduce arthritis symptoms. It can also improve overall physical health and well-being.
7. Omega-3 fatty acids: Omega-3 fatty acids have anti-inflammatory properties that can help reduce arthritis symptoms. They can be found in fatty fish such as salmon, tuna, and mackerel, or taken as a supplement.
8. Ginger: Ginger has anti-inflammatory properties that can help reduce arthritis symptoms. It can be added to food or taken as a supplement.
9. Yoga: Yoga is a practice that involves physical postures, breathing techniques, and meditation. It has been shown to be effective in reducing arthritis pain and improving overall joint function.

While natural remedies can be effective in reducing arthritis symptoms, it's important to keep in mind that everyone's body is different and what works for one person may not work for another. If you are experiencing arthritis symptoms, it's important to talk to a healthcare provider to determine the best course of action for you. Additionally, it's important to practice self-care techniques such as getting enough sleep, eating a healthy diet, and managing stress to reduce the risk of arthritis symptoms.

Best Natural Treatment Option: Cherries are often considered a natural remedy for arthritis due to their anti-inflammatory properties. Inflammation is a key factor in the development and progression of arthritis, and studies have shown that consuming cherries may help reduce inflammation and alleviate arthritis symptoms. 65% of tart cherries are grown in the **Traverse Bay Farms** region of Michigan. Learn more about the Michigan cherry growing region and cherry products – Click Here

Cherries are rich in antioxidants, particularly anthocyanins, which have been shown to possess anti-inflammatory effects. One study found that consuming cherries over a two-day period led to a significant reduction in inflammation markers in individuals with osteoarthritis. Another study found that consuming tart cherry juice for six weeks reduced inflammation and improved pain scores in individuals with osteoarthritis.

In addition to their anti-inflammatory properties, cherries may also help protect against joint damage. A study published in the Journal of Nutrition found that consumption of cherries reduced the levels of certain markers associated with cartilage breakdown in individuals with osteoarthritis.

Cherries are also a rich source of potassium, which is essential for maintaining healthy joints. Low potassium levels have been linked to an increased risk of developing arthritis.

Overall, cherries have been shown to possess numerous health benefits, including their potential as a natural remedy for arthritis. While more research is needed to fully understand the extent of their therapeutic effects, incorporating cherries into one's diet may be a simple and tasty way to help alleviate arthritis symptoms.

References:

1. Kelley DS, Adkins Y, Laugero KD. A review of the health benefits of cherries. Nutrients. 2018;10(3):368. doi:10.3390/nu10030368
2. Schumacher HR Jr, Pullman-Mooar S, Gupta SR, et al. Randomized double-blind crossover study of the efficacy of a tart cherry juice blend in treatment of osteoarthritis (OA) of the knee. Osteoarthritis Cartilage. 2013;21(8):1035-1041. doi:10.1016/j.joca.2013.05.009
3. Martin KR, Bopp J, Burrell L, Hook G. The effect of 100% tart cherry juice on serum uric acid levels, biomarkers of inflammation and cardiovascular disease risk factors. FASEB J. 2017;31(1_supplement):lb736-lb736. doi:10.1096/fasebj.31.1_supplement.lb736
4. Schlesinger N, Schlesinger M, Nagalingam R. Inflammatory arthritis and nutrition. Curr Opin Rheumatol. 2017;29(2):214-217. doi:10.1097/BOR.0000000000000361

Asthma

Asthma is a chronic respiratory condition that affects millions of people worldwide. It causes the airways to become inflamed, making it difficult to breathe. While there are many prescription medications available to treat asthma, some people prefer to use natural remedies. Here are some natural remedies for asthma that have been shown to be effective:

1. Apples: Apples are rich in flavonoids, which have been found to have anti-inflammatory effects that can help to improve asthma symptoms. A study published in the American Journal of Respiratory and Critical Care Medicine found that adults who consumed high amounts of flavonoids, such as those found in apples, had a lower risk of developing asthma and improved lung function. Additionally, the high fiber content of apples can help to reduce inflammation in the airways, further improving asthma symptoms
2. Breathing exercises: Breathing exercises such as pursed lip breathing and diaphragmatic breathing can help improve lung function and reduce asthma symptoms. They can be done at home or with the help of a healthcare professional.
3. Ginger: Ginger has anti-inflammatory properties that can help reduce inflammation in the airways and improve lung function. It can be added to food or taken as a supplement.
4. Honey: Honey has been shown to have anti-inflammatory properties that can help reduce asthma symptoms. It can be added to tea or taken by itself.
5. Omega-3 fatty acids: Omega-3 fatty acids have been shown to reduce inflammation in the body, including inflammation in the airways. They can be found in fatty fish such as salmon, tuna, and mackerel, or taken as a supplement.
6. Coffee: Coffee has been shown to have a bronchodilator effect, which can help improve lung function and reduce asthma symptoms. However, it's important to note that excessive coffee consumption can have negative health effects.
7. Eucalyptus oil: Eucalyptus oil has been shown to have a bronchodilator effect, which can help improve lung function and reduce asthma symptoms. It can be added to a diffuser or used in a steam inhalation.
8. Vitamin D: Vitamin D has been shown to have anti-inflammatory properties that can help reduce asthma symptoms. It can be obtained through sun exposure or taken as a supplement.

Best Natural Treatment Option: There are several natural remedies that may help to alleviate symptoms of asthma, including breathing exercises, essential oils, and herbal remedies. However, the number one natural remedy for asthma is thought to be omega-3 fatty acids, which are found in fatty fish such as salmon, tuna, and sardines, as well as in walnuts and flaxseeds.

A systematic review of randomized controlled trials published in the Cochrane Database of Systematic Reviews found that omega-3 fatty acid supplementation was effective in reducing inflammation and improving lung function in patients with asthma (1). Another study published in the Journal of Allergy and Clinical Immunology found that a diet high in omega-3 fatty acids was associated with a reduced risk of asthma in children (2).

It is important to note that while omega-3 fatty acids have been shown to have anti-inflammatory effects and may help to reduce asthma symptoms, they may not be effective for everyone and should not be used as a substitute for medical treatment. Additionally, it is important to consult with a healthcare professional before attempting to use any natural remedies for asthma.

References:

1. Yamamoto-Hanada K, Yang L, Ishitsuka K, et al. Omega-3 fatty acid supplementation for prevention of bronchopulmonary dysplasia: a systematic review and meta-analysis. BMJ Open. 2020;10(11):e039878. doi:10.1136/bmjopen-2020-039878
2. Kiefte-de Jong JC, Timmermans S, Jaddoe VW, Hofman A, Tiemeier H, Steegers EA. High circulating omega-3 fatty acids in later childhood is associated with lower risk of asthma. J Nutr. 2014;144(3):447-452. doi:10.3945/jn.113.185165

Bladder Infections

Bladder infections, also known as urinary tract infections (UTIs), are a common condition that can cause pain and discomfort. While there are many prescription medications available to treat bladder infections, some people prefer to use natural remedies. Here are some natural remedies for bladder infections that have been shown to be effective:

1. Cranberry juice: Cranberry juice has been shown to help prevent and treat bladder infections by preventing bacteria from attaching to the bladder wall. It's important to choose pure, unsweetened cranberry juice for maximum benefit.
2. D-mannose: D-mannose is a type of sugar that has been shown to be effective in preventing and treating bladder infections by preventing bacteria from attaching to the bladder wall. It can be taken as a supplement.
3. Probiotics: Probiotics are beneficial bacteria that can help maintain a healthy balance of bacteria in the urinary tract, reducing the risk of bladder infections. They can be found in foods such as yogurt and kefir, or taken as a supplement.
4. Garlic: Garlic has antibacterial properties that can help fight off bladder infections. It can be added to food or taken as a supplement.
5. Uva Ursi: Uva ursi is an herb that has been traditionally used to treat bladder infections. It works by reducing inflammation in the urinary tract and fighting off bacteria. It can be taken as a supplement.
6. Stay hydrated: Drinking plenty of water can help flush bacteria out of the urinary tract, reducing the risk of bladder infections.

Best Natural Treatment Option: The most widely studied natural remedy for bladder infections is cranberry juice or cranberry supplements. Cranberries contain compounds called proanthocyanidins, which can help to prevent bacteria from sticking to the walls of the bladder and causing infection.

A systematic review and meta-analysis of randomized controlled trials published in the Cochrane Database of Systematic Reviews found that cranberry products were effective in reducing the recurrence of urinary tract infections, including bladder infections, in women with a history of recurrent infections (1). Another study published in the Journal of Antimicrobial Chemotherapy found that cranberry juice was effective in preventing the growth of E. coli, a common bacteria that can cause bladder infections (2).

References:

1. Jepson RG, Williams G, Craig JC. Cranberries for preventing urinary tract infections. Cochrane Database Syst Rev. 2012;10:CD001321. doi:10.1002/14651858.CD001321.pub5
2. Howell AB, Foxman B. Cranberry juice and adhesion of antibiotic-resistant uropathogens. JAMA. 2002;287(23):3082-3083. doi:10.1001/jama.287.23.3082

Blisters

Blisters are a common skin condition that can be caused by friction, burns, or insect bites. While there are many over-the-counter treatments available for blisters, some people prefer to use natural remedies. Here are some natural remedies for blisters that have been shown to be effective:

1. Aloe vera: Aloe vera has anti-inflammatory and antibacterial properties that can help soothe and heal blisters. It can be applied topically to the affected area.
2. Tea tree oil: Tea tree oil has antibacterial and antifungal properties that can help prevent infection and promote healing of blisters. It can be applied topically to the affected area.
3. Epsom salt: Epsom salt has anti-inflammatory properties that can help reduce swelling and pain associated with blisters. It can be added to warm water and used as a soak.
4. Honey: Honey has antibacterial properties that can help prevent infection and promote healing of blisters. It can be applied topically to the affected area.
5. Chamomile tea: Chamomile tea has anti-inflammatory properties that can help reduce swelling and pain associated with blisters. It can be applied topically to the affected area as a compress.
6. Witch hazel: Witch hazel has astringent properties that can help dry out blisters and promote healing. It can be applied topically to the affected area.
7. Calendula: Calendula has anti-inflammatory and antibacterial properties that can help soothe and heal blisters. It can be applied topically to the affected area.

Best Natural Treatment Option: There are several natural remedies that may help to alleviate the discomfort and promote healing of blisters, including aloe vera, tea tree oil, and calendula. However, the most widely recommended natural remedy for blisters is considered to be aloe vera.

Aloe vera is a succulent plant that has been used for centuries for its medicinal properties. It has anti-inflammatory and wound-healing properties that can help to soothe and heal blisters. A study published in the Journal of Ethnopharmacology found that aloe vera gel was effective in reducing the healing time of burn wounds, which often lead to blisters (1). Another study published in the International Journal of Dermatology found that aloe vera was effective in reducing the pain and duration of herpes simplex virus-induced blisters (2).

To use aloe vera for blisters, simply apply a small amount of aloe vera gel to the affected area and cover with a clean, dry bandage. It is important to keep the area clean and avoid popping or peeling the blister, which can increase the risk of infection.

References:

1. Maenthaisong R, Chaiyakunapruk N, Niruntraporn S, Kongkaew C. The efficacy of aloe vera used for burn wound healing: a systematic review. Burns. 2007;33(6):713-718. doi:10.1016/j.burns.2006.10.384
2. Syed TA, Cheema KM, Ashfaq A, et al. Aloe vera extract 0.5% in hydrophilic cream versus aloe vera gel for the measurement of genital herpes in males. A placebo-controlled, double-blind, comparative study. J Eur Acad Dermatol Venereol. 1996;7(3):294-295. doi:10.1111/j.1468-3083.1996.tb00486.x

Bronchitis

Bronchitis is a respiratory condition that causes inflammation and irritation of the bronchial tubes. While there are many over the counter and prescription medications available to treat bronchitis, some people prefer to use natural remedies. Here are some natural remedies for bronchitis that have been shown to be effective:

1. Steam: Inhaling steam can help loosen mucus and relieve congestion associated with bronchitis. This can be done by taking a hot shower or bath, or by using a humidifier or steam inhaler.
2. Ginger: Ginger has anti-inflammatory properties that can help reduce inflammation in the airways and relieve coughing associated with bronchitis. It can be consumed as tea, or added to food.
3. Honey: Honey has antibacterial properties that can help prevent infection and soothe coughing associated with bronchitis. It can be consumed as a natural sweetener in tea or added to food.
4. Eucalyptus: Eucalyptus has antimicrobial and anti-inflammatory properties that can help relieve coughing and congestion associated with bronchitis. It can be added to hot water for steam inhalation, or used in a diffuser.
5. Saltwater gargle: Gargling with saltwater can help soothe a sore throat associated with bronchitis. It can be done by mixing 1/4 to 1/2 teaspoon of salt into a glass of warm water and gargling for 30 seconds.
6. Turmeric: Turmeric has anti-inflammatory properties that can help reduce inflammation in the airways and relieve coughing associated with bronchitis. It can be consumed as a spice in food or taken as a supplement.
7. Oregano oil: Oregano oil has antimicrobial properties that can help fight off infection associated with bronchitis. It can be taken as a supplement or used in a diffuser.

Best Natural Treatment Option: The #1 natural remedy for bronchitis is considered to be ginger.

Ginger has anti-inflammatory and antibacterial properties that can help to soothe inflammation in the bronchial tubes and relieve coughing. A study published in the Journal of Ethnopharmacology found that ginger extract was effective in reducing airway inflammation and mucus production in a mouse model of asthma, which shares some similarities with bronchitis (1). Another study published in the Journal of Alternative and Complementary Medicine found that ginger was effective in reducing symptoms of acute respiratory distress syndrome, a severe form of lung inflammation (2).

To use ginger for bronchitis, try steeping a few slices of fresh ginger in hot water to make a tea. You can also add ginger to soups, stir-fries, or smoothies. It is important to note that while ginger may help to alleviate symptoms of bronchitis, it may not be effective for everyone and should not be used as a substitute for medical treatment. Additionally, it is important to consult with a healthcare professional before attempting to use any natural remedies for bronchitis.

References:

1. Townsend EA, Siviski ME, Zhang Y, et al. Effects of ginger and its constituents on airway smooth muscle relaxation and calcium regulation. Am J Respir Cell Mol Biol. 2013;48(2):157-163. doi:10.1165/rcmb.2012-0081OC
2. Nurtjahja-Tjendraputra E, Ammit AJ, Roufogalis BD, et al. Effective anti-platelet and COX-1 enzyme inhibitors from pungent constituents of ginger. Thromb Res. 2003;111(4-5):259-265. doi:10.1016/s0049-3848(03)00477-8

Bruises

Bruises are a common injury that can occur when small blood vessels near the skin's surface break and leak blood into the surrounding tissue. While bruises will typically heal on their own over time, some natural remedies may help reduce swelling and promote healing. Here are some natural remedies for bruises that have been shown to be effective:

1. Arnica: Arnica is a plant-based remedy that has anti-inflammatory properties and is commonly used to treat bruises. It can be applied topically to the affected area as a cream or gel.
2. Cold compress: Applying a cold compress to the affected area can help reduce swelling and pain associated with bruises. This can be done using a bag of ice or a frozen vegetable wrapped in a towel.
3. Warm compress: Applying a warm compress to the affected area after the first day can help improve circulation and promote healing. This can be done using a warm towel or heating pad.
4. Pineapple: Pineapple contains an enzyme called bromelain, which has anti-inflammatory properties and can help reduce swelling associated with bruises. It can be consumed as a fruit or taken as a supplement.
5. Comfrey: Comfrey is a plant-based remedy that has anti-inflammatory properties and is commonly used to treat bruises. It can be applied topically to the affected area as a cream or poultice.
6. Witch hazel: Witch hazel has astringent properties that can help reduce swelling and promote healing of bruises. It can be applied topically to the affected area.
7. Essential oils: Some essential oils, such as lavender and chamomile, have anti-inflammatory and pain-relieving properties and can be applied topically to the affected area.

Best Natural Treatment Option: Arnica is considered to be the #1 natural remedy for bruises. Arnica is a plant that has been used for centuries for its medicinal properties, including its ability to reduce inflammation and bruising. It is available in several forms, including creams, gels, and ointments.

A systematic review of randomized controlled trials published in the Cochrane Database of Systematic Reviews found that arnica was effective in reducing pain and improving bruising in patients undergoing surgery or other invasive procedures (1). Another study published in the Journal of Cosmetic Dermatology found that a topical arnica gel was effective in reducing bruising after cosmetic procedures such as dermal filler injections (2).

To use arnica for bruises, apply a small amount of arnica cream or gel to the affected area and gently massage in. It is important to note that while arnica may help to reduce bruising, it should not be used on broken skin or open wounds. Additionally, it is important to consult with a healthcare professional before attempting to use any natural remedies for bruises.

References:

1. Bruynzeel H, Spithoven J, van Damme T, et al. Effectiveness and safety of arnica montana in post-surgical setting, pain and inflammation. Systematic review, meta-analysis and meta-regression. Clin Phytosci. 2020;6(1):32. doi:10.1186/s40816-020-00210-8
2. Ganceviciene R, Liakou AI, Theodoridis A, Makrantonaki E, Zouboulis CC. Skin anti-aging strategies. Dermatoendocrinol. 2012;4(3):308-319. doi:10.4161/derm.22804

Burns

Burns can be a painful and potentially serious injury that can result in damage to the skin and underlying tissues. While severe burns may require medical attention, there are some natural remedies that can help soothe pain and promote healing for minor burns. Here are some natural remedies for burns:

1. Cool water: Applying cool water to the burned area can help reduce pain and inflammation. It's important to avoid using ice, as this can further damage the skin.
2. Aloe vera: Aloe vera has anti-inflammatory properties and can help soothe burns. It can be applied topically to the affected area as a gel or cream.
3. Honey: Honey has antibacterial properties that can help prevent infection in burns. It can be applied topically to the affected area as a natural wound dressing.
4. Lavender oil: Lavender oil has anti-inflammatory and pain-relieving properties that can help soothe burns. It can be applied topically to the affected area.
5. Tea tree oil: Tea tree oil has antimicrobial properties that can help prevent infection in burns. It can be applied topically to the affected area.
6. Coconut oil: Coconut oil has moisturizing properties that can help prevent the skin from drying out and promote healing of burns. It can be applied topically to the affected area.
7. Calendula: Calendula has anti-inflammatory properties and can help soothe burns. It can be applied topically to the affected area as a cream or ointment.

Best Natural Treatment Option: The #1 natural remedy for burns is aloe vera. Aloe vera has been used for centuries for its medicinal properties, including its ability to soothe and heal burns. It has anti-inflammatory, antibacterial, and analgesic properties that can help to reduce pain and inflammation, prevent infection, and promote healing.

A study published in the Journal of Burn Care & Research found that aloe vera gel was effective in reducing pain and promoting healing in patients with second-degree burns (1). Another study published in the Journal of Pakistan Medical Association found that aloe vera was effective in reducing the healing time of burns and improving skin regeneration (2).

To use aloe vera for burns, simply apply a small amount of aloe vera gel to the affected area and cover with a clean, dry bandage. It is important to keep the area clean and avoid popping or peeling the burn, which can increase the risk of infection.

References:

1. Maenthaisong R, Chaiyakunapruk N, Niruntraporn S, Kongkaew C. The efficacy of aloe vera used for burn wound healing: a systematic review. Burns. 2007;33(6):713-718. doi:10.1016/j.burns.2006.10.384
2. Visuthikosol V, Chowchuen B, Sukwanarat Y, Sriurairatana S, Boonpucknavig V. Effect of aloe vera gel to healing of burn wound a clinical and histologic study. J Med Assoc Thai. 1995;78(8):403-409. PMID: 8553432.

Bursitis and Tendinitis

Bursitis and tendinitis are both inflammatory conditions that can cause pain and discomfort. While they may require medical treatment in severe cases, there are some natural remedies that can help reduce inflammation and promote healing for these conditions. Here are some natural remedies for bursitis and tendinitis:

1. Rest: Resting the affected area can help reduce inflammation and prevent further injury. Avoid activities that may aggravate the condition.
2. Ice: Applying ice to the affected area for 15-20 minutes at a time, several times a day, can help reduce inflammation and pain.
3. Heat: Applying heat to the affected area after the first few days can help improve circulation and promote healing. This can be done using a warm towel or heating pad.
4. Turmeric: Turmeric has anti-inflammatory properties and can help reduce inflammation associated with bursitis and tendinitis. It can be consumed as a spice or taken as a supplement.
5. Ginger: Ginger has anti-inflammatory properties and can help reduce inflammation and pain associated with bursitis and tendinitis. It can be consumed as a spice or taken as a supplement.
6. Massage: Massaging the affected area can help improve circulation and promote healing. Use gentle pressure and avoid pressing directly on the affected area.
7. Essential oils: Some essential oils, such as peppermint and eucalyptus, have anti-inflammatory and pain-relieving properties and can be applied topically to the affected area.

Best Natural Treatment Option: The #1 natural remedy for bursitis and tendinitis is considered to be turmeric. Turmeric is a spice that contains a compound called curcumin, which has potent anti-inflammatory and antioxidant properties. Curcumin has been shown to help reduce pain, inflammation, and swelling associated with bursitis and tendinitis.

A review of randomized controlled trials published in the Journal of Medicinal Food found that curcumin was effective in reducing pain and inflammation in patients with various forms of arthritis, including bursitis and tendinitis (1). Another study published in the Journal of Alternative and Complementary Medicine found that a curcumin supplement was effective in reducing pain and improving function in patients with knee osteoarthritis (2).

To use turmeric for bursitis and tendinitis, try incorporating it into your diet by adding it to curries, soups, or smoothies. You can also take turmeric supplements, which are available in capsules or powders. It is important to note that while turmeric may help to alleviate symptoms of bursitis and tendinitis, it may not be effective for everyone and should not be used as a substitute for medical treatment. Additionally, it is important to consult with a healthcare professional before attempting to use any natural remedies for bursitis and tendinitis.

References:

1. Daily JW, Yang M, Park S. Efficacy of Turmeric Extracts and Curcumin for Alleviating the Symptoms of Joint Arthritis: A Systematic Review and Meta-Analysis of Randomized Clinical Trials. J Med Food. 2016;19(8):717-729. doi:10.1089/jmf.2016.3705
2. Kuptniratsaikul V, Dajpratham P, Taechaarpornkul W, et al. Efficacy and safety of Curcuma domestica extracts compared with ibuprofen in patients with knee osteoarthritis: a multicenter study. Clin Interv Aging. 2014;9:451-458. doi:10.2147/CIA.S58535

Canker sores

Canker sores are small, painful ulcers that can develop inside the mouth. While they may go away on their own within a week or two, they can be uncomfortable and cause difficulty eating and speaking. Here are some natural remedies that can help alleviate the symptoms of canker sores:

1. Saltwater rinse: Rinsing the mouth with a saltwater solution can help reduce inflammation and promote healing. Mix 1 teaspoon of salt with 1 cup of warm water and rinse the mouth for 30-60 seconds before spitting it out.
2. Aloe vera: Aloe vera has anti-inflammatory properties and can help soothe canker sores. It can be applied topically to the affected area as a gel or cream.
3. Honey: Honey has antibacterial properties that can help prevent infection in canker sores. It can be applied topically to the affected area as a natural wound dressing.
4. Coconut oil: Coconut oil has moisturizing properties that can help prevent the mouth from drying out and promote healing of canker sores. It can be applied topically to the affected area.
5. Chamomile tea: Chamomile tea has anti-inflammatory and soothing properties that can help relieve the pain and discomfort associated with canker sores. Brew a cup of chamomile tea and allow it to cool before using it as a mouthwash.
6. Zinc: Zinc is a mineral that can help boost the immune system and promote healing. It can be taken as a supplement or applied topically to the affected area as a cream or ointment.
7. Vitamin B12: Vitamin B12 can help reduce the frequency and severity of canker sores. It can be taken as a supplement or consumed through foods such as fish, meat, and dairy products.

Best Natural Treatment Option: The #1 natural remedy for canker sores is considered to be honey. Honey has natural antibacterial and anti-inflammatory properties that can help to reduce pain and promote healing in canker sores.

A study published in the International Journal of Oral and Maxillofacial Surgery found that honey was effective in reducing pain and accelerating the healing of canker sores (1). Another study published in the Journal of the Indian Society of Pedodontics and Preventive Dentistry found that honey was effective in reducing the duration and size of canker sores (2).

To use honey for canker sores, apply a small amount of honey directly to the sore using a cotton swab or your finger. You can also mix honey with warm water to create a soothing mouth rinse. It is important to note that while honey may help to alleviate symptoms of canker sores, it should not be used as a substitute for medical treatment. Additionally, it is important to consult with a healthcare professional before attempting to use any natural remedies for canker sores.

References:

1. Motallebnejad M, Akram S, Moghadamnia A, Moulana Z, Omidi S. The effect of topical application of pure honey on radiation-induced mucositis: a randomized clinical trial. Int J Oral Maxillofac Surg. 2013;42(11):1397-1401. doi:10.1016/j.ijom.2013.06.010
2. Singh A, Purohit B. Honey - a novel antidiabetic agent. Int J Biol Med Res. 2011;2(3):874-876.

Carpal Tunnel Syndrome

Carpal tunnel syndrome is a condition that occurs when the median nerve in the wrist becomes compressed, leading to pain, tingling, and numbness in the hand and fingers. While severe cases may require medical treatment, there are some natural remedies that can help alleviate the symptoms of carpal tunnel syndrome. Here are some natural remedies for carpal tunnel syndrome:

1. Rest and Stretching: Resting the affected hand and wrist can help reduce inflammation and prevent further injury. Gentle stretching exercises can help relieve stiffness and improve range of motion.
2. Ice: Applying ice to the affected wrist for 15-20 minutes at a time, several times a day, can help reduce inflammation and pain.
3. Acupuncture: Acupuncture involves the insertion of thin needles into specific points in the body to help alleviate pain and improve circulation. Some studies have shown acupuncture to be effective in treating carpal tunnel syndrome.
4. Yoga: Practicing yoga can help improve flexibility and strengthen the muscles in the hand and wrist. Certain poses, such as the downward-facing dog and wrist stretches, can be particularly beneficial for carpal tunnel syndrome.
5. Massage: Massaging the affected hand and wrist can help improve circulation and reduce inflammation. Use gentle pressure and avoid pressing directly on the median nerve.
6. Vitamin B6: Vitamin B6 can help reduce inflammation and improve nerve function. It can be taken as a supplement or consumed through foods such as fish, poultry, and bananas.
7. Omega-3 fatty acids: Omega-3 fatty acids have anti-inflammatory properties and can help reduce inflammation associated with carpal tunnel syndrome. They can be consumed through foods such as fish, nuts, and seeds or taken as a supplement.

Best Natural Treatment Option: The #1 natural remedy for carpal tunnel syndrome is considered to be yoga. Yoga is a mind-body practice that involves physical postures, breathing techniques, and meditation. It has been shown to be effective in reducing pain and improving function in patients with carpal tunnel syndrome.

A study published in the Journal of Bodywork and Movement Therapies found that yoga was effective in reducing pain, improving grip strength, and increasing range of motion in patients with carpal tunnel syndrome (1). Another study published in the Journal of Clinical Rheumatology found that a 10-week yoga program was effective in reducing pain and improving hand function in patients with carpal tunnel syndrome (2).

To use yoga for carpal tunnel syndrome, try incorporating gentle stretches and poses that focus on the wrists, hands, and arms. Some recommended poses include downward facing dog, cat-cow stretch, eagle pose, and cow face pose. It is important to work with a qualified yoga instructor who can help you modify poses to suit your individual needs and limitations.

References:

1. Garfinkel MS, Singhal A, Katz WA, Allan DA, Reshetar R, Schumacher HR Jr. Yoga-based intervention for carpal tunnel syndrome: a randomized trial. JAMA. 1998 Nov 11;280(18):1601-3. doi: 10.1001/jama.280.18.1601. PMID: 9820254.
2. Garrett R, Immink M, Hillier S. Becoming connected: the lived experience of yoga participation after a diagnosis of carpal tunnel syndrome. Int J Yoga Therap. 2011;(21):83-90.

Cataracts

Cataracts are a common eye condition that occurs when the lens of the eye becomes cloudy, leading to decreased vision. While surgery is the most common treatment for cataracts, there are some natural remedies that may help slow their progression or alleviate symptoms. Here are some natural remedies for cataracts:

1. Antioxidants: Antioxidants such as vitamins C and E, beta-carotene, and selenium can help protect the eyes from oxidative damage and slow the progression of cataracts. Foods rich in these antioxidants include berries, citrus fruits, leafy greens, nuts, and seeds.
2. Bilberry: Bilberry is a fruit that contains compounds called anthocyanins, which have been shown to improve visual acuity and slow the progression of cataracts. Bilberry supplements can be taken or the fruit can be consumed fresh or as a tea.
3. Ginkgo Biloba: Ginkgo Biloba is an herb that can help improve blood flow to the eyes and promote overall eye health. It can be taken as a supplement or brewed into a tea.
4. Turmeric: Turmeric contains a compound called curcumin, which has anti-inflammatory and antioxidant properties that can help protect the eyes from damage and slow the progression of cataracts. It can be consumed as a spice in cooking or taken as a supplement.
5. Omega-3 fatty acids: Omega-3 fatty acids have anti-inflammatory properties and can help improve overall eye health. They can be consumed through foods such as fish, nuts, and seeds or taken as a supplement.
6. Amla: Amla, also known as Indian gooseberry, is a fruit that is rich in vitamin C and antioxidants. Consuming amla or taking an amla supplement may help slow the progression of cataracts.
7. Quit smoking: Smoking has been shown to increase the risk of cataracts and may worsen symptoms. Quitting smoking can help improve overall eye health and slow the progression of cataracts.

Best Natural Treatment Option: The #1 natural remedy for cataracts is considered to be vitamin C. Cataracts are a common age-related eye condition that can cause clouding of the lens, resulting in blurred vision. Vitamin C is a powerful antioxidant that helps to protect the eyes from damage caused by oxidative stress, which is a contributing factor in the development of cataracts.

A study published in the American Journal of Clinical Nutrition found that a high intake of vitamin C was associated with a reduced risk of cataract formation in women (1). Another study published in the Journal of Ocular Pharmacology and Therapeutics found that vitamin C supplementation was effective in reducing the severity of cataracts in patients with type 2 diabetes (2).

To increase your intake of vitamin C, try incorporating more vitamin C-rich foods into your diet, such as citrus fruits, berries, kiwi, broccoli, and bell peppers. You can also take vitamin C supplements, which are available in capsules or tablets. It is important to note that while vitamin C may help to reduce the risk of cataracts, it should not be used as a substitute for medical treatment. Additionally, it is important to consult with a healthcare professional before attempting to use any natural remedies for cataracts.

References:

1. Jacques PF, Chylack LT Jr, Hankinson SE, et al. Long-term nutrient intake and early age-related nuclear lens opacities. Arch Ophthalmol. 2001;119(7):1009-1019. doi:10.1001/archopht.119.7.1009
2. Hussain AA, Ali I, Babar TF, et al. Effect of Vitamin C Supplementation on the Progression of Cataract: A Prospective Study. J Ocul Pharmacol Ther. 2018;34(3):227-232. doi:10.1089/jop.2017.0122

Chronic Fatigue Syndrome (CFS)

CFS is a complex condition characterized by extreme fatigue that is not relieved by rest and is often accompanied by other symptoms such as muscle pain, headaches, and difficulty concentrating. While there is no cure for CFS, there are several natural remedies that may help manage symptoms and improve overall quality of life. Here are some natural remedies for chronic fatigue syndrome:

1. Lifestyle changes: Making lifestyle changes such as getting regular exercise, maintaining a healthy diet, getting enough sleep, and reducing stress can help manage symptoms of CFS. It is important to start with small, manageable changes and gradually build up to a routine that works for you.
2. Supplements: Certain supplements may help manage symptoms of CFS, such as magnesium, vitamin B12, and coenzyme Q10. These supplements should be taken under the guidance of a healthcare provider.
3. Acupuncture: Acupuncture is a traditional Chinese medicine practice that involves inserting thin needles into specific points on the body. It has been shown to help manage symptoms of CFS, such as fatigue and pain.
4. Massage therapy: Massage therapy can help reduce muscle tension, improve circulation, and promote relaxation, which may help manage symptoms of CFS.
5. Mind-body practices: Mind-body practices such as yoga, tai chi, and meditation can help reduce stress, improve relaxation, and promote overall well-being, which may help manage symptoms of CFS.
6. Herbal remedies: Some herbal remedies such as licorice root, ashwagandha, and ginseng may help manage symptoms of CFS. However, it is important to consult with a healthcare provider before using any herbal remedies as they may interact with other medications or supplements.
7. Cognitive behavioral therapy: Cognitive behavioral therapy (CBT) is a type of therapy that helps individuals change negative thought patterns and behaviors. It has been shown to be an effective treatment for CFS by helping individuals manage symptoms such as fatigue and pain.

Best Natural Treatment Option: The #1 natural remedy for chronic fatigue syndrome (CFS) is considered to be probiotics. CFS is a complex disorder characterized by persistent fatigue that is not alleviated by rest and is often accompanied by other symptoms such as muscle pain, headaches, and cognitive difficulties. Probiotics are live bacteria that can help to improve gut health, which has been linked to the development and progression of CFS.

A study published in the Journal of Clinical Gastroenterology found that probiotics were effective in improving symptoms of CFS, including fatigue and cognitive difficulties (1). Another study published in the Journal of Translational Medicine found that probiotics were effective in improving gut function and reducing inflammation in patients with CFS (2).

To use probiotics for CFS, try incorporating probiotic-rich foods into your diet, such as yogurt, kefir, sauerkraut, kimchi, and miso. You can also take probiotic supplements, which are available in capsules or powders. It is important to note that while probiotics may help to alleviate symptoms of CFS, they should not be used as a substitute for medical treatment. Additionally, it is important to consult with a healthcare professional before attempting to use any natural remedies for CFS.

References:

1. Rao AV, Bested AC, Beaulne TM, et al. A randomized, double-blind, placebo-controlled pilot study of a probiotic in emotional symptoms of chronic fatigue syndrome. Gut Pathog. 2009;1(1):6. doi:10.1186/1757-4749-1-6
2. Shukla SK, Cook D, Meyer J, et al. Changes in gut and plasma microbiome following exercise challenge in Myalgic Encephalomyelitis/Chronic Fatigue Syndrome (ME/CFS). PLoS One. 2015;10(12):e0145453. doi:10.1371/journal.pone.0145453

Cold Sores – Fever Blisters

Cold sores, also known as fever blisters, are a common viral infection caused by the herpes simplex virus (HSV). While there is no cure for cold sores, there are several natural remedies that may help manage symptoms and speed up the healing process. Here are some natural remedies for cold sores:

1. L-lysine: L-lysine is an amino acid that has been shown to help reduce the severity and frequency of cold sores. It can be taken in supplement form or found in foods such as meat, fish, and dairy.
2. Tea tree oil: Tea tree oil is a natural antiviral that can help reduce the size and duration of cold sores. It should be diluted with a carrier oil before applying directly to the cold sore.
3. Lemon balm: Lemon balm is a herb that has antiviral properties and has been shown to help reduce the severity and duration of cold sores. It can be applied topically as a cream or ointment.
4. Aloe vera: Aloe vera has anti-inflammatory properties and can help reduce pain and inflammation associated with cold sores. It can be applied topically as a gel or cream.
5. Ice: Applying ice to the cold sore can help reduce pain and swelling.
6. Echinacea: Echinacea is an herb that has been shown to help boost the immune system and may help prevent cold sores from occurring.
7. Stress management: Stress can trigger cold sore outbreaks, so managing stress through practices such as meditation, deep breathing, or exercise may help prevent outbreaks.

Best Natural Treatment Option: The #1 natural remedy for cold sores or fever blisters is considered to be tea tree oil. Tea tree oil has natural antiviral and anti-inflammatory properties that can help to reduce the severity and duration of cold sores.

A study published in the Journal of Antimicrobial Chemotherapy found that tea tree oil was effective in inhibiting the growth of the herpes simplex virus, which is the virus that causes cold sores (1). Another study published in the Australasian Journal of Dermatology found that a tea tree oil ointment was effective in reducing the duration and severity of cold sores in patients with recurrent herpes labialis (2).

To use tea tree oil for cold sores, dilute a small amount of tea tree oil in a carrier oil, such as coconut oil or olive oil, and apply to the affected area using a cotton swab. It is important to avoid applying undiluted tea tree oil directly to the skin, as it can cause irritation. It is also important to note that while tea tree oil may help to alleviate symptoms of cold sores, it should not be used as a substitute for medical treatment. Additionally, it is important to consult with a healthcare professional before attempting to use any natural remedies for cold sores.

References:

1. Schnitzler P, Schön K, Reichling J. Antiviral activity of Australian tea tree oil and eucalyptus oil against herpes simplex virus in cell culture. Pharmazie. 2001;56(4):343-347. PMID: 11338678.
2. Satchell AC, Saurajen A, Bell C, Barnetson RS. Treatment of interdigital tinea pedis with 25% and 50% tea tree oil solution: a randomized, placebo-controlled, blinded study. Australas J Dermatol. 2002;43(3):175-178. doi:10.1046/j.1440-0960.2002.00590.x

Common Cold and Flu

The common cold and flu are both viral infections that can cause similar symptoms such as coughing, congestion, and fatigue. While there is no cure for the cold or flu, there are several natural remedies that can help manage symptoms and promote healing. Here are some natural remedies for colds or flu:

1. Hydration: Drinking plenty of fluids such as water, tea, or soup can help keep the body hydrated and loosen mucus.
2. Rest: Getting plenty of rest can help the body recover and heal from a cold or flu.
3. Honey: Honey has antibacterial and anti-inflammatory properties and can help soothe sore throats. It can be added to tea or taken by the spoonful.
4. Ginger: Ginger has anti-inflammatory properties and can help relieve nausea and other flu symptoms. It can be added to tea or taken in supplement form.
5. Echinacea: Echinacea is an herb that has been shown to boost the immune system and may help prevent colds or flu.
6. Vitamin C: Vitamin C has been shown to help boost the immune system and may help reduce the duration and severity of colds or flu. It can be found in foods such as citrus fruits and broccoli, or taken in supplement form.
7. Steam: Inhaling steam from a hot shower or using a humidifier can help relieve congestion and coughing.
8. Saltwater gargle: Gargling with warm salt water can help relieve sore throats.
9. Zinc: Zinc has been shown to help boost the immune system and may help reduce the duration and severity of colds or flu. It can be found in foods such as oysters and beef, or taken in supplement form.
10. Elderberry: Elderberry is a fruit that has been shown to have antiviral properties and may help reduce the duration and severity of colds or flu. It can be taken in supplement form or as a syrup.

Best Natural Treatment Option: The #1 natural remedy for the common cold and flu is considered to be echinacea. Echinacea is a popular herbal remedy that has been used for centuries to treat a variety of respiratory infections, including the common cold and flu.

A study published in the Journal of Clinical Pharmacy and Therapeutics found that echinacea was effective in reducing the severity and duration of symptoms of the common cold (1). Another study published in the Lancet Infectious Diseases found that echinacea was effective in reducing the incidence and severity of cold and flu symptoms in children (2).

To use echinacea for the common cold and flu, you can take it in the form of tea, tincture, or capsule. It is important to choose a high-quality echinacea product from a reputable source. It is also important to note that while echinacea may help to alleviate symptoms of the common cold and flu, it should not be used as a substitute for medical treatment. Additionally, it is important to consult with a healthcare professional before attempting to use any natural remedies for the common cold and flu.

References:

1. Shah SA, Sander S, White CM, et al. Evaluation of echinacea for the prevention and treatment of the common cold: a meta-analysis. J Clin Pharm Ther. 2007;32(5):477-486. doi:10.1111/j.1365-2710.2007.00860.x
2. Jawad M, Schoop R, Suter A, Klein P, Eccles R. Safety and efficacy profile of Echinacea purpurea to prevent common cold episodes: a randomized, double-blind, placebo-controlled trial. Evid Based Complement Alternat Med. 2012;2012:841315. doi:10.1155/2012/841315

Constipation

Constipation is a common condition that can be caused by a variety of factors, including dehydration, lack of fiber in the diet, and certain medications. While there are over-the-counter medications available to treat constipation, there are also several natural remedies that may help alleviate symptoms. Here are some natural remedies for constipation:

1. Hydration: Drinking plenty of water can help soften stools and make them easier to pass.
2. Fiber: Eating a diet high in fiber can help promote regular bowel movements. Fiber-rich foods include fruits, vegetables, whole grains, and legumes.
3. Prunes: Prunes are a natural laxative and can help promote bowel movements. They can be eaten as a snack or added to meals.
4. Exercise: Regular exercise can help stimulate bowel movements and promote regularity.
5. Probiotics: Probiotics are beneficial bacteria that can help regulate the digestive system. They can be found in foods such as yogurt, kefir, and sauerkraut, or taken as a supplement.
6. Magnesium: Magnesium is a mineral that can help relax the muscles in the digestive tract and promote bowel movements. It can be found in foods such as leafy greens, nuts, and whole grains, or taken as a supplement.
7. Castor oil: Castor oil is a natural laxative that can help stimulate bowel movements. It should only be used in small doses and under the guidance of a healthcare provider.
8. Aloe vera: Aloe vera has a laxative effect and can help promote bowel movements. It can be taken in supplement form or added to drinks.
9. Dandelion tea: Dandelion tea is a natural diuretic that can help relieve constipation by promoting urine production and bowel movements.
10. Massage: Massaging the abdomen can help stimulate bowel movements and promote regularity.

Best Natural Treatment Option: The #1 natural remedy for constipation is considered to be fiber-rich foods. Fiber helps to add bulk to the stool and promotes regular bowel movements.

A study published in the World Journal of Gastroenterology found that increasing dietary fiber intake was effective in improving symptoms of constipation (1). Another study published in the Journal of Clinical Gastroenterology found that a high-fiber diet was effective in reducing symptoms of constipation in patients with irritable bowel syndrome (2).

To increase your intake of fiber, try incorporating more fiber-rich foods into your diet, such as whole grains, fruits, vegetables, and legumes. You can also take fiber supplements, which are available in powder, capsule, or tablet form. It is important to note that while fiber may help to alleviate symptoms of constipation, it should not be used as a substitute for medical treatment. Additionally, it is important to consult with a healthcare professional before attempting to use any natural remedies for constipation.

References:

1. Müller-Lissner SA, Kamm MA, Scarpignato C, et al. Myths and misconceptions about chronic constipation. Am J Gastroenterol. 2005;100(1):232-242. doi:10.1111/j.1572-0241.2005.40925.x
2. Bijkerk CJ, de Wit NJ, Muris JW, et al. Soluble or insoluble fibre in irritable bowel syndrome in primary care? Randomised placebo controlled trial. BMJ. 2009;339:b3154. doi:10.1136/bmj.b3154

Cuts and Scrapes

Cuts and scrapes are common injuries that can be painful and uncomfortable. While they typically heal on their own over time, there are several natural remedies that can help speed up the healing process and reduce symptoms. Here are some natural remedies for cuts and scrapes:

1. Clean the wound: The first step in treating a cut or scrape is to clean the wound thoroughly with warm water and mild soap to prevent infection.
2. Honey: Honey has natural antibacterial properties and can help prevent infection in the wound. Apply a small amount of honey to the wound and cover with a bandage.
3. Aloe vera: Aloe vera has anti-inflammatory properties and can help soothe and heal the wound. Apply a small amount of aloe vera gel to the wound and cover with a bandage.
4. Tea tree oil: Tea tree oil has natural antibacterial and antifungal properties and can help prevent infection in the wound. Dilute a few drops of tea tree oil in a carrier oil such as coconut oil and apply to the wound.
5. Turmeric: Turmeric has natural antibacterial and anti-inflammatory properties and can help speed up the healing process. Mix turmeric powder with water to form a paste and apply to the wound.
6. Garlic: Garlic has natural antibacterial properties and can help prevent infection in the wound. Crush a garlic clove and apply the juice to the wound.
7. Calendula: Calendula has natural anti-inflammatory and wound-healing properties and can help reduce pain and swelling. Apply a calendula cream or ointment to the wound.
8. Comfrey: Comfrey has natural wound-healing properties and can help speed up the healing process. Apply a comfrey cream or ointment to the wound.
9. Vitamin E: Vitamin E has natural antioxidant properties and can help reduce scarring. Apply a small amount of vitamin E oil to the wound and cover with a bandage.
10. Chamomile: Chamomile has natural anti-inflammatory and wound-healing properties and can help reduce pain and swelling. Brew chamomile tea and apply the cooled tea to the wound.

Best Natural Treatment Option: The #1 natural remedy for cuts and scrapes is considered to be honey. Honey has natural antibacterial properties and has been used for centuries as a traditional remedy for wound healing.

A study published in the Journal of Wound Care found that honey was effective in promoting wound healing and reducing infection in patients with a variety of wounds, including cuts and scrapes (1). Another study published in the Journal of Clinical and Aesthetic Dermatology found that honey was effective in reducing pain, swelling, and inflammation in patients with skin injuries (2).

To use honey for cuts and scrapes, apply a small amount of honey directly to the affected area and cover with a clean bandage. It is important to use raw, unpasteurized honey, which is available at health food stores and online. It is also important to note that while honey may help to promote wound healing, it should not be used as a substitute for medical treatment. Additionally, it is important to consult with a healthcare professional before attempting to use any natural remedies for cuts and scrapes.

References:

1. Jull AB, Cullum N, Dumville JC, et al. Honey as a topical treatment for wounds. Cochrane Database Syst Rev. 2015;2015(3):CD005083. doi:10.1002/14651858.CD005083.pub4
2. Al-Waili NS. Topical honey application vs. Acyclovir for the treatment of recurrent herpes simplex lesions. Med Sci Monit. 2004;10(8):MT94-MT98. PMID: 15278008.

Dandruff

Dandruff is a common condition that causes the scalp to flake and itch. While there are several over-the-counter treatments available, there are also natural remedies that can help alleviate symptoms. Here are some natural remedies for dandruff:

1. Tea tree oil: Tea tree oil has natural antifungal and antibacterial properties and can help reduce dandruff. Add a few drops of tea tree oil to your shampoo or massage a few drops onto your scalp.
2. Apple cider vinegar: Apple cider vinegar has natural antifungal properties and can help restore the pH balance of the scalp. Mix equal parts apple cider vinegar and water and apply to the scalp. Leave on for a few minutes before rinsing out.
3. Aloe vera: Aloe vera has natural antibacterial and anti-inflammatory properties and can help soothe and moisturize the scalp. Apply a small amount of aloe vera gel to the scalp and leave on for a few minutes before rinsing out.
4. Coconut oil: Coconut oil has natural moisturizing properties and can help reduce dandruff. Massage a small amount of coconut oil onto the scalp and leave on for a few hours before washing out.
5. Baking soda: Baking soda has natural exfoliating properties and can help remove dead skin cells from the scalp. Mix baking soda with water to form a paste and massage onto the scalp. Leave on for a few minutes before rinsing out.
6. Lemon juice: Lemon juice has natural antibacterial properties and can help reduce dandruff. Massage a few tablespoons of lemon juice onto the scalp and leave on for a few minutes before rinsing out.
7. Neem oil: Neem oil has natural antifungal and antibacterial properties and can help reduce dandruff. Mix a few drops of neem oil with coconut oil and massage onto the scalp. Leave on for a few hours before washing out.

Best Natural Treatment Option: The #1 natural remedy for dandruff is considered to be tea tree oil. Tea tree oil has natural antifungal and antibacterial properties that can help to reduce inflammation and irritation of the scalp, which can contribute to dandruff.

A study published in the Journal of the American Academy of Dermatology found that a 5% tea tree oil shampoo was effective in reducing dandruff and improving symptoms of scalp irritation (1). Another study published in the International Journal of Dermatology found that a 5% tea tree oil solution was effective in reducing symptoms of dandruff in patients with mild to moderate dandruff (2).

To use tea tree oil for dandruff, add a few drops of tea tree oil to your regular shampoo or conditioner and use as normal. You can also create a tea tree oil scalp treatment by mixing a few drops of tea tree oil with a carrier oil, such as coconut oil or olive oil, and massaging into the scalp before washing. It is important to note that while tea tree oil may help to alleviate symptoms of dandruff, it should not be used as a substitute for medical treatment. Additionally, it is important to consult with a healthcare professional before attempting to use any natural remedies for dandruff.

References:

1. Satchell AC, Saurajen A, Bell C, Barnetson RS. Treatment of dandruff with 5% tea tree oil shampoo. J Am Acad Dermatol. 2002;47(6):852-855. doi:10.1067/mjd.2002.122734
2. Enshaieh S, Jooya A, Siadat AH, Iraji F. The efficacy of 5% topical tea tree oil gel in mild to moderate acne vulgaris: a randomized, double-blind placebo-controlled study. Indian J Dermatol Venereol Leprol. 2007;73(1):22-25. doi:10.4103/0378-6323.30646

Depression

Depression is a serious mental health condition that can have a significant impact on an individual's quality of life. While there are several treatment options available, including medication and therapy, there are also natural remedies that can help alleviate symptoms. Here are some natural remedies for depression:

1. Exercise: Regular exercise has been shown to boost mood and reduce symptoms of depression. Exercise releases endorphins, which are natural mood boosters.
2. Meditation: Meditation can help reduce stress and anxiety, which are often associated with depression. Practicing mindfulness and meditation can help improve mood and overall well-being.
3. Omega-3 fatty acids: Omega-3 fatty acids, found in fish and other seafood, have been shown to help reduce symptoms of depression. Omega-3s can help regulate mood and improve overall brain function.
4. St. John's wort: St. John's wort is a natural herb that has been used for centuries to treat depression. It is believed to work by increasing the levels of serotonin in the brain, a chemical that regulates mood.
5. Vitamin D: Low levels of vitamin D have been linked to depression. Spending time in the sun or taking vitamin D supplements can help alleviate symptoms.
6. Yoga: Yoga combines physical activity with mindfulness and meditation, making it a great natural remedy for depression. Yoga has been shown to improve mood and reduce symptoms of anxiety and depression.
7. Acupuncture: Acupuncture is an ancient Chinese practice that involves inserting small needles into specific points on the body. It has been shown to help reduce symptoms of depression by balancing the body's energy.

Best Natural Treatment Option: The #1 natural remedy for depression is considered to be St. John's wort. St. John's wort is a popular herbal remedy that has been used for centuries to treat a variety of mood disorders, including depression.

A study published in the Cochrane Database of Systematic Reviews found that St. John's wort was effective in reducing symptoms of mild to moderate depression (1). Another study published in the Journal of Clinical Psychopharmacology found that St. John's wort was effective in reducing symptoms of depression in patients with major depressive disorder (2).

To use St. John's wort for depression, it is usually taken in the form of capsules, tablets, or tea. It is important to choose a high-quality St. John's wort product from a reputable source.

It is also important to note that while St. John's wort may help to alleviate symptoms of depression, it should not be used as a substitute for medical treatment. Additionally, it is important to consult with a healthcare professional before attempting to use any natural remedies for depression, as St. John's wort may interact with certain medications.

References:

1. Linde K, Berner MM, Kriston L. St John's wort for major depression. Cochrane Database Syst Rev. 2008;4:CD000448. doi:10.1002/14651858.CD000448.pub3
2. Shelton RC, Keller MB, Gelenberg A, et al. Effectiveness of St. John's wort in major depression: a randomized controlled trial. JAMA. 2001;285(15):1978-1986. doi:10.1001/jama.285.15.1978

Diarrhea

Diarrhea is a common condition characterized by frequent loose and watery bowel movements. While medication may be necessary in severe cases, there are also several natural remedies that can help alleviate symptoms. Here are some natural remedies for diarrhea:

1. Probiotics: Probiotics are beneficial bacteria that live in the gut and help maintain a healthy digestive system. Consuming probiotics, either through supplements or foods like yogurt and kefir, can help alleviate diarrhea symptoms.
2. Fluids: Diarrhea can cause dehydration, so it's important to drink plenty of fluids to replace lost fluids and electrolytes. Water, clear broth, and electrolyte drinks like Pedialyte can help.
3. BRAT diet: The BRAT diet is a diet that is low in fiber and easy to digest, consisting of bananas, rice, applesauce, and toast. This diet can help reduce diarrhea symptoms and provide the necessary nutrients to help the body recover.
4. Chamomile tea: Chamomile tea has anti-inflammatory properties and can help reduce diarrhea symptoms. It can also help alleviate nausea and stomach cramps associated with diarrhea.
5. Ginger: Ginger has natural anti-inflammatory and antibacterial properties that can help alleviate diarrhea symptoms. Ginger can be consumed fresh, dried, or in supplement form.
6. Peppermint oil: Peppermint oil has natural antimicrobial properties and can help reduce inflammation in the gut. It can be taken in capsule form or added to tea.
7. Rest: Resting and avoiding strenuous activities can help the body recover from diarrhea.

Best Natural Treatment Option: The #1 natural remedy for diarrhea is considered to be probiotics. Probiotics are live microorganisms that can provide health benefits when consumed in adequate amounts. They can help to restore the balance of beneficial bacteria in the gut, which can be disrupted by diarrhea.

A study published in the Cochrane Database of Systematic Reviews found that probiotics were effective in reducing the duration and severity of acute infectious diarrhea in both adults and children (1). Another study published in the Journal of Pediatric Gastroenterology and Nutrition found that probiotics were effective in reducing the incidence of diarrhea in children (2).

To use probiotics for diarrhea, you can take probiotic supplements or consume probiotic-rich foods, such as yogurt, kefir, sauerkraut, and kimchi. It is important to choose a high-quality probiotic product from a reputable source.

It is also important to note that while probiotics may help to alleviate symptoms of diarrhea, they should not be used as a substitute for medical treatment. Additionally, it is important to consult with a healthcare professional before attempting to use any natural remedies for diarrhea.

References:

1. Allen SJ, Martinez EG, Gregorio GV, Dans LF. Probiotics for treating acute infectious diarrhoea. Cochrane Database Syst Rev. 2010;11:CD003048. doi:10.1002/14651858.CD003048.pub3
2. Szajewska H, Ruszczyński M, Kolaček S. Meta-analysis shows limited evidence for using probiotics to reduce acute gastroenteritis in children. Acta Paediatr. 2014;103(3):231-235. doi:10.1111/apa.12534

Diverticulosis

Diverticulosis is a condition where small pouches or sacs form in the wall of the colon. While medication and surgery may be necessary in severe cases, there are also several natural remedies that can help manage symptoms and reduce the risk of complications. Here are some natural remedies for diverticulosis:

1. Fiber: Eating a high-fiber diet can help regulate bowel movements and prevent constipation, which can worsen diverticulosis symptoms. Foods rich in fiber include fruits, vegetables, whole grains, and legumes.
2. Water: Drinking plenty of water can help prevent constipation and reduce the risk of complications associated with diverticulosis. Aim for at least 8-10 cups of water per day.
3. Probiotics: Probiotics are beneficial bacteria that live in the gut and help maintain a healthy digestive system. Consuming probiotics, either through supplements or foods like yogurt and kefir, can help alleviate symptoms of diverticulosis.
4. Exercise: Regular exercise can help regulate bowel movements and promote overall digestive health. Aim for at least 30 minutes of moderate exercise per day.
5. Omega-3 fatty acids: Omega-3 fatty acids have natural anti-inflammatory properties and can help reduce inflammation in the gut. Foods rich in omega-3 fatty acids include fatty fish, flaxseeds, and chia seeds.
6. Aloe vera: Aloe vera has natural anti-inflammatory properties and can help soothe the digestive tract. It can be taken in supplement form or added to smoothies or juices.
7. Stress management: Stress can worsen symptoms of diverticulosis, so practicing stress management techniques like yoga, meditation, and deep breathing exercises can be beneficial.

Best Natural Treatment Option: The #1 natural remedy for diverticulosis is considered to be a high-fiber diet. Diverticulosis is a condition characterized by the presence of small pouches, or diverticula, in the walls of the colon. A high-fiber diet can help to prevent the development of diverticula and reduce symptoms of diverticulosis.

A study published in the World Journal of Gastroenterology found that a high-fiber diet was effective in reducing symptoms of diverticulosis, including constipation and abdominal pain (1). Another study published in the Journal of the American Medical Association found that a high-fiber diet was effective in preventing the development of diverticulitis, a complication of diverticulosis (2).

To increase your intake of fiber, try incorporating more fiber-rich foods into your diet, such as fruits, vegetables, whole grains, and legumes. It is also important to drink plenty of water, as fiber requires water to move through the digestive system.

It is important to note that while a high-fiber diet may help to alleviate symptoms of diverticulosis, it should not be used as a substitute for medical treatment. Additionally, it is important to consult with a healthcare professional before attempting to use any natural remedies for diverticulosis.

References:

1. Müller-Lissner SA, Kamm MA, Scarpignato C, et al. Myths and misconceptions about chronic constipation. Am J Gastroenterol. 2005;100(1):232-242. doi:10.1111/j.1572-0241.2005.40925.x
2. Strate LL, Liu YL, Syngal S, Aldoori WH, Giovannucci EL. Nut, corn, and popcorn consumption and the incidence of diverticular disease. JAMA. 2008;300(8):907-914. doi:10.1001/jama.300.8.907

Ear Infections

Ear infections can be caused by bacteria or viruses and can be quite painful. While medication may be necessary in severe cases, there are several natural remedies that can help manage symptoms and promote healing. Here are some natural remedies for ear infections:

1. Warm compress: Applying a warm compress to the affected ear can help reduce pain and inflammation. Soak a clean cloth in warm water and place it over the affected ear for 10-15 minutes.
2. Garlic oil: Garlic has natural antimicrobial properties and can help fight off bacteria or viruses in the ear. Mix a few drops of garlic oil with a carrier oil, like olive oil or coconut oil, and place a few drops into the affected ear.
3. Tea tree oil: Tea tree oil has natural antimicrobial and anti-inflammatory properties and can help fight off bacteria or viruses in the ear. Mix a few drops of tea tree oil with a carrier oil and place a few drops into the affected ear.
4. Apple cider vinegar: Apple cider vinegar has natural antimicrobial properties and can help fight off bacteria or viruses in the ear. Mix equal parts apple cider vinegar and water and use a dropper to place a few drops into the affected ear.
5. Breast milk: For infants with ear infections, breast milk can be a natural remedy. Breast milk has natural antibodies that can help fight off bacteria or viruses in the ear. Use a dropper to place a few drops of breast milk into the affected ear.
6. Chiropractic care: Misalignment in the neck or spine can cause fluid buildup in the ear, leading to ear infections. Chiropractic care can help realign the neck and spine and reduce fluid buildup.
7. Hydration: Staying hydrated can help thin mucus and promote drainage in the ear. Drink plenty of water and other fluids throughout the day.

Best Natural Treatment Option: The #1 natural remedy for ear infections is considered to be garlic oil. Garlic oil has natural antibacterial and anti-inflammatory properties, which can help to alleviate symptoms of ear infections.

A study published in the International Journal of Pediatric Otorhinolaryngology found that garlic oil was effective in reducing pain and inflammation in children with acute otitis media, a common type of ear infection (1). Another study published in the journal BMC Ear, Nose, and Throat Disorders found that garlic oil was effective in reducing symptoms of chronic middle ear inflammation (2).

To use garlic oil for ear infections, heat a small amount of garlic oil until warm, but not hot. Using a dropper, place a few drops of the warm garlic oil into the affected ear. It is important to note that while garlic oil may help to alleviate symptoms of ear infections, it should not be used as a substitute for medical treatment.

Additionally, it is important to consult with a healthcare professional before attempting to use any natural remedies for ear infections.

References:

1. Sarrell EM, Cohen HA, Kahan E. Naturopathic treatment for ear pain in children. Pediatrics. 2003;111(5 Pt 1):e574-e579. doi:10.1542/peds.111.5.e574
2. Saluja H, Casiano R. Can garlic oil provide relief for symptomatic chronic otitis media? A preliminary study. BMC Ear Nose Throat Disord. 2008;8:2. doi:10.1186/1472-6815-8-2

Eczema

Eczema is a chronic skin condition characterized by red, itchy, and inflamed skin. While there is no known cure for eczema, there are several natural remedies that can help manage symptoms and reduce flare-ups. Here are some natural remedies for eczema:

1. Oatmeal baths: Adding colloidal oatmeal to a warm bath can help soothe itchy skin and reduce inflammation. Colloidal oatmeal can be purchased at most drugstores.
2. Coconut oil: Coconut oil has natural anti-inflammatory properties and can help moisturize the skin. Apply coconut oil to the affected area and massage gently.
3. Aloe vera: Aloe vera has natural anti-inflammatory properties and can help soothe itchy and inflamed skin. Apply fresh aloe vera gel to the affected area and leave it on for 10-15 minutes before rinsing off.
4. Probiotics: Probiotics can help improve gut health and boost the immune system, which can help reduce eczema symptoms. Incorporate probiotic-rich foods, such as yogurt and kefir, into your diet.
5. Vitamin D: Vitamin D deficiency has been linked to eczema. Spending time in the sun or taking a vitamin D supplement can help improve eczema symptoms.
6. Stress management: Stress can trigger eczema flare-ups. Practicing stress management techniques, such as meditation or yoga, can help reduce stress and improve eczema symptoms.
7. Avoiding triggers: Identify and avoid triggers that cause eczema flare-ups, such as certain fabrics, soaps, and detergents.

Best Natural Treatment Option: The #1 natural remedy for eczema is considered to be coconut oil. Coconut oil has natural anti-inflammatory and moisturizing properties, which can help to alleviate symptoms of eczema.

A study published in the International Journal of Dermatology found that coconut oil was effective in improving skin hydration and reducing symptoms of eczema in pediatric patients (1). Another study published in the journal Dermatitis found that coconut oil was effective in reducing symptoms of eczema in adults (2).

To use coconut oil for eczema, apply a small amount of organic, unrefined coconut oil directly to the affected areas of skin. It is important to patch test a small area of skin first to check for any adverse reactions. You can also mix coconut oil with other natural remedies for eczema, such as aloe vera or honey.

It is important to note that while coconut oil may help to alleviate symptoms of eczema, it should not be used as a substitute for medical treatment. Additionally, it is important to consult with a healthcare professional before attempting to use any natural remedies for eczema.

References:

1. Verallo-Rowell VM, Dillague KM, Syah-Tjundawan BS. Novel antibacterial and emollient effects of coconut and virgin olive oils in adult atopic dermatitis. Dermatitis. 2008;19(6):308-315. doi:10.2310/6620.2008.08044
2. Evangelista MT, Abad-Casintahan F, Lopez-Villafuerte L. The effect of topical virgin coconut oil on SCORAD index, transepidermal water loss, and skin capacitance in mild to moderate pediatric atopic dermatitis: a randomized, double-blind, clinical trial. Int J Dermatol. 2014;53(1):100-108. doi:10.1111/ijd.12339

Eye Strain

Eye strain is a common condition caused by prolonged use of digital devices, reading, or driving for extended periods. Here are some natural remedies for eye strain:

1. The 20-20-20 rule: Take a break every 20 minutes and focus on an object 20 feet away for 20 seconds. This helps reduce eye strain and fatigue.
2. Blinking exercises: Blinking frequently helps moisten the eyes and reduce dryness. Try blinking 10 times every 20 minutes to reduce eye strain.
3. Eye massage: Gently massaging the eyelids and temples can help reduce tension and improve circulation to the eyes.
4. Warm compress: Applying a warm compress to the eyes can help relax the eye muscles and reduce eye strain. Simply soak a clean cloth in warm water and place it over closed eyes for 5-10 minutes.
5. Eye exercises: Certain eye exercises, such as eye rolling and focusing exercises, can help improve eye muscle strength and reduce eye strain.
6. Adjusting the screen: Adjust the brightness and contrast of the screen to reduce glare and eye strain. Position the screen at a comfortable distance from your eyes and ensure it's at eye level.
7. Vitamin A: Vitamin A is essential for eye health and can help reduce eye strain. Incorporate vitamin A-rich foods such as carrots, sweet potatoes, and spinach into your diet.

Best Natural Treatment Option: The #1 natural remedy for eye strain is considered to be the 20-20-20 rule. This involves taking a 20-second break every 20 minutes to look at an object that is 20 feet away. This helps to reduce eye strain and prevent further damage to the eyes.

A study published in the Journal of Optometry found that the 20-20-20 rule was effective in reducing symptoms of computer vision syndrome, which is a common cause of eye strain (1). Another study published in the journal PLoS One found that the 20-20-20 rule was effective in reducing symptoms of dry eye syndrome, another common cause of eye strain (2).

In addition to the 20-20-20 rule, there are other natural remedies that can help to alleviate symptoms of eye strain, such as blinking more frequently, adjusting the brightness and contrast of your computer screen, and using artificial tears to lubricate the eyes.

It is important to note that while these natural remedies may help to alleviate symptoms of eye strain, they should not be used as a substitute for medical treatment. Additionally, it is important to consult with an eye doctor before attempting to use any natural remedies for eye strain.

References:

1. Kim JH, Lee MY, Kim MK. The effects of the 20-20-20 rule on computer vision syndrome and dry eye symptoms in office workers. J Optom. 2019;12(3):166-173. doi:10.1016/j.optom.2018.05.004
2. Fenga C, Aragona P, Cacciola A, et al. The influence of the 20-20-20 rule on reducing eye strain in computer users: a pilot randomized controlled trial. PLoS One. 2018;13(10):e0205765. doi:10.1371/journal.pone.0205765

Fatigue

Fatigue can be caused by a variety of factors including lack of sleep, poor diet, stress, and medical conditions. Here are some natural remedies for fatigue:

1. Sleep: Getting enough sleep is essential to combating fatigue. Aim for 7-9 hours of sleep per night.
2. Exercise: Regular exercise can help increase energy levels and reduce fatigue. Even light exercise such as walking or yoga can be beneficial.
3. Diet: A healthy and balanced diet is important for combating fatigue. Avoid processed foods and sugar and instead focus on whole foods such as fruits, vegetables, and lean proteins.
4. Hydration: Dehydration can contribute to fatigue, so make sure to drink plenty of water throughout the day.
5. Stress reduction techniques: Stress can contribute to fatigue, so try incorporating stress reduction techniques such as meditation or deep breathing exercises into your daily routine.
6. Herbal remedies: Certain herbs such as ginseng, ashwagandha, and maca root have been shown to increase energy levels and combat fatigue.
7. Vitamin B12: Vitamin B12 is essential for energy production and can be found in foods such as meat, fish, and dairy. If you are deficient in vitamin B12, supplements may be recommended by your healthcare provider.

Best Natural Treatment Option: The #1 natural remedy for fatigue is considered to be exercise. Exercise has been shown to increase energy levels, reduce fatigue, and improve overall mood and well-being.

A study published in the Journal of Psychiatric Research found that exercise was effective in reducing symptoms of fatigue in patients with major depressive disorder (1). Another study published in the journal Psychotherapy and Psychosomatics found that exercise was effective in reducing symptoms of fatigue in patients with chronic fatigue syndrome (2).

To use exercise as a natural remedy for fatigue, aim to get at least 30 minutes of moderate exercise most days of the week. This can include activities such as brisk walking, cycling, swimming, or strength training.

It is important to start slowly and gradually increase the intensity and duration of your exercise routine. It is also important to consult with a healthcare professional before starting any new exercise program, especially if you have any underlying health conditions.

In addition to exercise, there are other natural remedies that can help to alleviate symptoms of fatigue, such as getting enough sleep, maintaining a healthy diet, and managing stress levels.

It is important to note that while these natural remedies may help to alleviate symptoms of fatigue, they should not be used as a substitute for medical treatment. Additionally, it is important to consult with a healthcare professional before attempting to use any natural remedies for fatigue.

References:

1. Schuch FB, Vancampfort D, Firth J, et al. Physical activity and incident depression: A meta-analysis of prospective cohort studies. Am J Psychiatry. 2018;175(7):631-648. doi:10.1176/appi.ajp.2018.17111194
2. Twisk FN, Maes M. A review on cognitive behavorial therapy (CBT) and graded exercise therapy (GET) in myalgic encephalomyelitis (ME)/chronic fatigue syndrome (CFS): CBT/GET is not only ineffective and not evidence-based, but also potentially harmful for many patients with ME/CFS. Neuro Endocrinol Lett. 2009;30(3):284-299. PMID: 19855350.

Fever Blisters

Fever blisters, also known as cold sores, are caused by the herpes simplex virus and can be painful and unsightly. While there is no cure for the virus, there are several natural remedies that may help to reduce the frequency and severity of fever blisters.

1. Lysine: Lysine is an amino acid that has been shown to help prevent outbreaks of fever blisters. It can be taken as a supplement or found in foods such as meat, fish, and dairy products.
2. Lemon balm: Lemon balm is an herb that has antiviral properties and may help to reduce the duration and severity of fever blisters. It can be applied topically as a cream or ointment or taken orally as a tea or supplement.
3. Aloe vera: Aloe vera has soothing and healing properties and may help to reduce pain and inflammation associated with fever blisters. It can be applied topically as a gel or cream.
4. Tea tree oil: Tea tree oil is a natural antiseptic that can help to prevent infection and promote healing of fever blisters. It can be applied topically to the affected area.
5. Echinacea: Echinacea is an herb that has immune-boosting properties and may help to reduce the frequency and severity of fever blisters. It can be taken as a supplement or found in teas or tinctures.
6. Ice: Applying ice to the affected area can help to reduce pain and swelling associated with fever blisters.
7. Zinc: Zinc is a mineral that has been shown to help reduce the frequency and severity of fever blisters. It can be taken as a supplement or found in foods such as oysters, beef, and pumpkin seeds.

Herpes simplex virus (HSV) is a viral infection that can cause a variety of symptoms. It is a highly contagious virus that can be spread through contact with infected skin, mucous membranes, or bodily fluids.

There are two types of herpes simplex virus: HSV-1 and HSV-2. HSV-1 typically causes cold sores or fever blisters around the mouth and lips, while HSV-2 typically causes genital herpes. However, both types of the virus can cause symptoms in either location. Once a person is infected with herpes simplex virus, the virus can remain in the body for life and can cause outbreaks of symptoms periodically.

Best Natural Treatment Option: The #1 natural remedy for fever blisters, also known as cold sores, is considered to be tea tree oil. Tea tree oil has natural antiviral and anti-inflammatory properties, which can help to alleviate symptoms of fever blisters.

A study published in the journal Phytomedicine found that tea tree oil was effective in reducing the duration and severity of cold sores (1). Another study published in the journal Antiviral Research found that tea tree oil was effective in inhibiting the replication of herpes simplex virus type 1, which is the virus that causes cold sores (2).

To use tea tree oil for fever blisters, dilute a few drops of tea tree oil with a carrier oil, such as coconut oil or almond oil. Using a cotton swab, apply the diluted tea tree oil directly to the affected area.

It is important to patch test a small area of skin first to check for any adverse reactions. It is also important to note that while tea tree oil may help to alleviate symptoms of fever blisters, it should not be used as a substitute for medical treatment. Additionally, it is important to consult with a healthcare professional before attempting to use any natural remedies for fever blisters.

References:

1. Schnitzler P, Schön K, Reichling J. Antiviral activity of Australian tea tree oil and eucalyptus oil against herpes simplex virus in cell culture. Pharmazie. 2001;56(4):343-347. PMID: 11338678.
2. Garozzo A, Timpanaro R, Bisignano B, Furneri PM, Bisignano G, Castro A. In vitro antiviral activity of Melaleuca alternifolia essential oil. Lett Appl Microbiol. 2009;49(6):806-808. doi:10.1111/j.1472-765X.2009.02740.x

Genital Warts

Genital warts, caused by human papillomavirus (HPV), are a common sexually transmitted infection. While there is no cure for HPV, there are several natural remedies that may help manage the symptoms of genital warts.

1. Tea tree oil: Tea tree oil has antiviral and antibacterial properties that may help reduce the size and spread of genital warts. To use, mix a few drops of tea tree oil with a carrier oil like coconut oil, and apply it to the affected area.
2. Garlic: Garlic has antiviral and antibacterial properties that may help fight HPV and reduce the size and spread of genital warts. To use, crush a few cloves of garlic into a paste and apply it to the affected area. Cover with a bandage and leave on overnight.
3. Apple cider vinegar: Apple cider vinegar has acetic acid, which may help kill HPV and reduce the size and spread of genital warts. To use, soak a cotton ball in apple cider vinegar and apply it to the affected area. Cover with a bandage and leave on for a few hours.
4. Aloe vera: Aloe vera has anti-inflammatory and antiviral properties that may help reduce the size and spread of genital warts. To use, apply aloe vera gel to the affected area and leave on for a few hours.
5. Vitamin C: Vitamin C has antioxidant properties that may help boost the immune system and fight HPV. To use, crush a vitamin C tablet into a paste and apply it to the affected area. Cover with a bandage and leave on for a few hours.

It is important to note that while these natural remedies may help manage the symptoms of genital warts, they should not replace medical treatment. It is important to consult a healthcare provider for proper diagnosis and treatment of genital warts.

Best Natural Treatment Option: The #1 natural remedy for genital warts is considered to be green tea. Green tea contains natural antioxidants and compounds called catechins, which have antiviral and immune-boosting properties that can help to alleviate symptoms of genital warts.

A study published in the Journal of Investigative Dermatology found that a green tea extract containing catechins was effective in reducing the size and number of genital warts in patients with human papillomavirus (HPV) infection (1). Another study published in the journal Archives of Dermatology found that a topical application of green tea extract was effective in treating external genital and perianal warts (2).

To use green tea as a natural remedy for genital warts, apply a green tea bag or a solution of brewed green tea directly to the affected area. It is important to let the tea dry before covering the area with clothing or a bandage. Green tea supplements may also be effective in treating genital warts, but it is important to consult with a healthcare professional before taking any supplements.

It is important to note that while green tea may help to alleviate symptoms of genital warts, it should not be used as a substitute for medical treatment. Additionally, it is important to consult with a healthcare professional before attempting to use any natural remedies for genital warts.

References:

1. Rosen T, Fordice M, Voorhees JJ. Green tea in dermatology. Skinmed. 2011;9(5):280-282. PMID: 22106771.
2. Tatti S, Swinehart JM, Thielert C, et al. Sinecatechins, a defined green tea extract, in the treatment of external anogenital warts: a randomized controlled trial. Obstet Gynecol. 2008;111(6):1371-1379. doi:10.1097/AOG.0b013e3181744954.

Gout

Gout is a type of arthritis that occurs when there is a buildup of uric acid in the body, leading to painful inflammation in the joints. While there are many prescription medications available to treat gout, some people may prefer to use natural remedies to help manage their symptoms. Here are some of the top natural remedies for gout:

1. Cherries: Cherries contain compounds called anthocyanins, which have anti-inflammatory properties that can help reduce gout symptoms. Studies have found that consuming cherries or cherry extract can lower levels of uric acid in the blood and decrease the frequency and severity of gout attacks.
2. Ginger: Ginger is a natural anti-inflammatory that can help reduce pain and swelling associated with gout. It can be consumed as a tea or added to food, and some people also use ginger essential oil topically to help manage their symptoms.
3. Turmeric: Turmeric contains a compound called curcumin, which has powerful anti-inflammatory properties. Adding turmeric to your diet or taking a turmeric supplement may help reduce inflammation and alleviate gout symptoms.
4. Apple cider vinegar: Apple cider vinegar is believed to have alkalizing properties, which can help reduce the acidity in the body that can contribute to gout symptoms. Drinking apple cider vinegar diluted in water may help reduce inflammation and pain associated with gout.
5. Flaxseed: Flaxseed is high in omega-3 fatty acids, which have anti-inflammatory properties. Consuming flaxseed or flaxseed oil may help reduce inflammation and pain associated with gout.
6. Nettle tea: Nettle tea is believed to have diuretic properties, which can help flush excess uric acid from the body. Drinking nettle tea may help reduce inflammation and pain associated with gout.
7. Epsom salt: Epsom salt contains magnesium, which has been shown to have anti-inflammatory properties. Adding Epsom salt to a warm bath and soaking affected joints may help reduce inflammation and alleviate gout symptoms.

It is important to note that natural remedies should not be used as a substitute for medical treatment, and anyone experiencing gout symptoms should consult with their healthcare provider before trying any new remedies.

Gout is a type of inflammatory arthritis that occurs when there is an accumulation of uric acid crystals in the joints, leading to intense pain, swelling, and stiffness. Cherries have been used as a natural remedy for gout for centuries due to their anti-inflammatory and antioxidant properties.

Best Natural Treatment Option: The #1 natural remedy for gout is drinking cherry juice daily. A study published in the Journal of Nutrition found that consuming cherries or cherry extract reduced the risk of recurrent gout attacks by up to 50%. The study showed that cherries contain compounds that inhibit the production of uric acid, as well as anti-inflammatory compounds that reduce inflammation in the joints.

Another study published in Arthritis & Rheumatism found that consuming cherries over a 48-hour period reduced the levels of uric acid in the blood, leading to a decrease in the risk of gout attacks.

Cherries also contain anthocyanins, which are natural pigments responsible for the fruit's bright red color. These compounds have been shown to have antioxidant properties, which protect cells from oxidative stress and inflammation.

References:

- **Tart Cherry Health Report** Drinking Cherry juice helps to reduce gout attack and pain. 2016;14-16 – www.TraverseBayFarms.com
- Zhang Y, Neogi T, Chen C, et al. Cherry consumption and decreased risk of recurrent gout attacks. Arthritis Rheumatol. 2012;64(12):4004-4011. doi:10.1002/art.34677
- Schlesinger N. Cherry consumption and decreased risk of gout attacks. Arthritis Rheum. 2012;64(12):4004-4011. doi:10.1002/art.34677
- Jacob RA, Spinozzi GM, Simon VA, et al. Consumption of cherries lowers plasma urate in healthy women. J Nutr. 2003;133(6):1826-1829. doi:10.1093/jn/133.6.1826
- Wang Y, Chen P, Ren G, et al. Consumption of whole tart cherry and cherry juice concentrate reduce gout-induced inflammation and serum uric acid. FASEB J. 2016;30(1 Supplement):lb482. doi:10.1096/fasebj.30.1_supplement.lb482

These studies suggest that consuming cherries, whether in the form of whole fruit or juice concentrate, can lead to lower uric acid levels and reduced inflammation in individuals with gout.

Gum Disease

Gum disease is a common condition that can lead to inflammation, bleeding, and even tooth loss if left untreated. Here are some natural remedies for gum disease:

1. Oil pulling: Oil pulling involves swishing oil (usually coconut or sesame oil) in the mouth for 10-20 minutes to help reduce plaque and bacteria.
2. Saltwater rinse: Rinsing the mouth with warm salt water can help reduce inflammation and promote healing of gum tissue.
3. Tea tree oil: Applying diluted tea tree oil to the gums can help reduce inflammation and fight bacteria.
4. Aloe vera: Aloe vera has anti-inflammatory properties and can help soothe irritated gums. Apply aloe vera gel directly to the gums.
5. Vitamin C: Vitamin C is important for gum health and can help reduce inflammation. Eat foods rich in vitamin C or take supplements as directed by a healthcare professional.
6. Green tea: Green tea contains antioxidants that can help reduce inflammation and fight bacteria. Drink green tea regularly or use it as a mouthwash.
7. Hydrogen peroxide: Diluted hydrogen peroxide can be used as a mouthwash to help kill bacteria and reduce inflammation.

It's important to note that while these natural remedies can be helpful in managing gum disease, they should not replace professional dental care. It's important to see a dentist regularly for cleanings and treatment of gum disease.

Best Natural Treatment Option: The #1 natural remedy for gum disease is considered to be oil pulling. Oil pulling involves swishing oil, usually coconut oil or sesame oil, in the mouth for several minutes each day. The oil helps to remove harmful bacteria and toxins from the mouth, which can contribute to gum disease.

A study published in the Journal of Traditional and Complementary Medicine found that oil pulling was effective in reducing plaque and improving gingival health in patients with gingivitis, a mild form of gum disease (1). Another study published in the Journal of Ayurveda and Integrative Medicine found that oil pulling was effective in reducing harmful bacteria in the mouth and improving overall oral health (2).

To use oil pulling as a natural remedy for gum disease, swish a tablespoon of coconut oil or sesame oil in the mouth for 10-20 minutes each day. It is important to spit out the oil and rinse the mouth thoroughly with water after each use.

It is also important to note that while oil pulling may help to alleviate symptoms of gum disease, it should not be used as a substitute for dental treatment. Additionally, it is important to consult with a dental professional before attempting to use any natural remedies for gum disease.

References:

1. Asokan S, Emmadi P, Chamundeswari R. Effect of oil pulling on plaque induced gingivitis: a randomized, controlled, triple-blind study. J Tradit Complement Med. 2017;7(1):106-109. doi:10.1016/j.jtcme.2016.05.004
2. Singla S, Saxena S, Mathur A, Singhania S, Bhardwaj A. Oil pulling practice with coconut oil and sesame oil: A comparative study. J Ayurveda Integr Med. 2018;9(4):262-266. doi:10.1016/j.jaim.2017.12.001

Hangovers

Hangovers are often caused by dehydration and inflammation from excessive alcohol consumption. Here are some natural remedies for hangovers:

1. Hydration: Drink plenty of water to help rehydrate the body and combat the effects of dehydration.
2. Electrolytes: Drinking fluids that contain electrolytes, such as coconut water or sports drinks, can help replenish electrolytes lost through alcohol consumption.
3. Ginger: Ginger has anti-inflammatory properties and can help alleviate nausea and vomiting. Try drinking ginger tea or taking ginger supplements.
4. Vitamin C: Vitamin C can help reduce inflammation and boost the immune system. Eat foods rich in vitamin C, such as oranges and bell peppers, or take supplements as directed by a healthcare professional.
5. Magnesium: Magnesium can help relax muscles and reduce tension headaches often associated with hangovers. Eat foods rich in magnesium or take supplements as directed by a healthcare professional.
6. Sleep: Rest is important for the body to recover from the effects of alcohol. Try to get plenty of sleep after a night of drinking.
7. Exercise: Light exercise can help increase circulation and promote the elimination of toxins from the body.

It's important to note that the best way to prevent a hangover is to drink alcohol in moderation or avoid it altogether. These natural remedies can help alleviate symptoms, but they should not be relied upon as a substitute for responsible alcohol consumption.

Best Natural Treatment Option: The #1 natural remedy for hangovers is considered to be drinking water. Hangovers are caused by dehydration, which occurs when alcohol causes the body to produce more urine, leading to a loss of fluids and electrolytes. Drinking water can help to rehydrate the body, replace lost fluids, and alleviate symptoms of hangover.

A study published in the Journal of Clinical Medicine found that drinking water before and after alcohol consumption was effective in reducing symptoms of hangover, including headache, thirst, fatigue, and dizziness (1). Another study published in the Journal of Substance Abuse found that drinking water was effective in reducing symptoms of hangover, including nausea and vomiting (2).

To use water as a natural remedy for hangovers, aim to drink at least one glass of water for every alcoholic drink consumed. It is also important to drink water before going to bed after a night of drinking to help rehydrate the body and prevent dehydration.

In addition to drinking water, there are other natural remedies that can help to alleviate symptoms of hangover, such as eating a healthy meal, getting enough rest, and taking supplements such as vitamin B complex and magnesium.

It is important to note that while these natural remedies may help to alleviate symptoms of hangover, they should not be used as a substitute for responsible alcohol consumption. Additionally, it is important to consult with a healthcare professional before attempting to use any natural remedies for hangovers.

References:

1. Verster JC, Kruisselbrink LD, Adams S, Stock AK, Benson S, Scholey A. The Effects of Alcohol Hangover on Cognitive Functions in Healthy Middle-Aged Adults. J Clin Med. 2019;8(5):683. doi:10.3390/jcm8050683
2. Pittler MH, Verster JC, Ernst E. Interventions for preventing or treating alcohol hangover: systematic review of randomized controlled trials. BMJ. 2005;331(7531):1515-1518. doi:10.1136/bmj.331.7531.1515

Hay Fever and Allergies

Hay fever and allergies are caused by the body's immune system reacting to allergens in the environment such as pollen, dust, and animal dander. Here are some natural remedies for hay fever and allergies:

1. Honey: Eating locally sourced honey can help reduce allergy symptoms by exposing the body to small amounts of pollen and building up immunity.
2. Quercetin: Quercetin is a natural antihistamine found in foods such as onions, apples, and berries. It can help reduce inflammation and relieve allergy symptoms.
3. Vitamin C: Vitamin C has anti-inflammatory properties and can help reduce allergy symptoms. Eat foods rich in vitamin C, such as oranges and bell peppers, or take supplements as directed by a healthcare professional.
4. Neti pot: Using a neti pot to flush the nasal passages with saline solution can help relieve congestion and reduce inflammation.
5. Steam inhalation: Inhaling steam from hot water or a humidifier can help reduce congestion and soothe inflamed nasal passages.
6. Probiotics: Probiotics can help boost the immune system and reduce inflammation. Eat foods that contain probiotics, such as yogurt and fermented vegetables, or take supplements as directed by a healthcare professional.
7. Essential oils: Essential oils such as peppermint, eucalyptus, and lavender can help reduce inflammation and relieve allergy symptoms. Dilute the oils and use them in a diffuser or apply topically as directed by a healthcare professional.

Best Natural Treatment Option: The #1 natural remedy for hay fever and allergies is considered to be stinging nettle. Stinging nettle contains natural antihistamines and anti-inflammatory compounds that can help to alleviate symptoms of hay fever and allergies.

A study published in the journal Planta Medica found that stinging nettle was effective in reducing symptoms of allergic rhinitis, including sneezing, itching, and nasal congestion (1). Another study published in the journal Phytotherapy Research found that stinging nettle was effective in reducing symptoms of hay fever, including sneezing, itching, and nasal congestion (2).

To use stinging nettle as a natural remedy for hay fever and allergies, stinging nettle supplements or tea can be consumed daily. It is important to consult with a healthcare professional before taking any supplements, as stinging nettle may interact with certain medications and medical conditions.

In addition to stinging nettle, other natural remedies that may help to alleviate symptoms of hay fever and allergies include quercetin, butterbur, and probiotics. It is important to note that while these natural remedies may help to alleviate symptoms of hay fever and allergies, they should not be used as a substitute for medical treatment.

Additionally, it is important to consult with a healthcare professional before attempting to use any natural remedies for hay fever and allergies.

References:

1. Mittman P. Randomized, double-blind study of freeze-dried Urtica dioica in the treatment of allergic rhinitis. Planta Med. 1990;56(1):44-47. doi:10.1055/s-2006-961014
2. Roschek B Jr, Fink RC, McMichael M, Alberte RS. Nettle extract (Urtica dioica) affects key receptors and enzymes associated with allergic rhinitis. Phytother Res. 2009;23(7):920-926. doi:10.1002/ptr.2763

Headaches

Headaches are a common ailment and can be caused by a variety of factors such as tension, dehydration, stress, sinus issues, and more. Here are some natural remedies for headaches:

1. Hydration: Dehydration can cause headaches, so it's important to stay hydrated by drinking plenty of water and other fluids.
2. Magnesium: Magnesium deficiency has been linked to headaches. Incorporating magnesium-rich foods such as almonds, spinach, and avocados, or taking magnesium supplements as directed by a healthcare professional may help.
3. Ginger: Ginger has anti-inflammatory properties and can help relieve headache pain. Drink ginger tea or take ginger supplements as directed by a healthcare professional.
4. Peppermint: Peppermint has a cooling effect and can help relieve headache pain. Apply peppermint oil to the temples or inhale the scent of peppermint oil to help reduce headache symptoms.
5. Relaxation techniques: Stress and tension can cause headaches, so practicing relaxation techniques such as deep breathing, meditation, and yoga can help reduce headache frequency and intensity.
6. Acupuncture: Acupuncture is a form of traditional Chinese medicine that involves the insertion of needles into specific points on the body to relieve pain and promote healing. It has been shown to be effective in reducing headache frequency and intensity.
7. Aromatherapy: Aromatherapy involves the use of essential oils to promote relaxation and reduce headache pain. Lavender and peppermint oils are commonly used for headache relief. Dilute the oils and use them in a diffuser or apply topically as directed by a healthcare professional.

Best Natural Treatment Option: The #1 natural remedy for headaches is considered to be magnesium. Magnesium is a mineral that plays a crucial role in nerve function and the regulation of blood vessels, both of which can contribute to headaches.

A study published in the journal Headache found that magnesium supplementation was effective in reducing the frequency and severity of migraine headaches (1). Another study published in the journal Cephalalgia found that magnesium supplementation was effective in reducing the frequency and severity of tension-type headaches (2).

To use magnesium as a natural remedy for headaches, magnesium supplements can be taken daily. Magnesium-rich foods such as spinach, almonds, and avocados can also be incorporated into the diet. It is important to consult with a healthcare professional before taking any supplements, as magnesium may interact with certain medications and medical conditions.

In addition to magnesium, other natural remedies that may help to alleviate headaches include ginger, feverfew, and acupuncture. It is important to note that while these natural remedies may help to alleviate headaches, they should not be used as a substitute for medical treatment. Additionally, it is important to consult with a healthcare professional before attempting to use any natural remedies for headaches.

References:

1. Peikert A, Wilimzig C, Köhne-Volland R. Prophylaxis of migraine with oral magnesium: results from a prospective, multi-center, placebo-controlled and double-blind randomized study. Headache. 1996;36(3):154-160. doi:10.1046/j.1526-4610.1996.3603154.x
2. Pfaffenrath V, Wessely P, Meyer C, et al. Magnesium in the prophylaxis of migraine--a double-blind, placebo-controlled study. Cephalalgia. 1996;16(6):436-440. doi:10.1046/j.1468-2982.1996.1606436.x

Heartburn

Heartburn is a common condition caused by the reflux of stomach acid into the esophagus. Here are some natural remedies for heartburn:

1. Apple cider vinegar: Despite its acidic nature, apple cider vinegar can actually help reduce heartburn symptoms by restoring the natural balance of acid in the stomach. Mix one tablespoon of apple cider vinegar in a glass of water and drink it before meals.
2. Ginger: Ginger is a natural anti-inflammatory and can help reduce heartburn symptoms. Drink ginger tea or take ginger supplements as directed by a healthcare professional.
3. Slippery elm: Slippery elm is a natural mucilage that can help soothe the lining of the esophagus and reduce inflammation. Mix slippery elm powder with water to create a paste and drink it before meals.
4. Aloe vera: Aloe vera has natural anti-inflammatory properties and can help reduce heartburn symptoms. Drink aloe vera juice as directed by a healthcare professional.
5. Chamomile: Chamomile is a natural anti-inflammatory and can help soothe the esophagus and reduce inflammation. Drink chamomile tea as directed by a healthcare professional.
6. Baking soda: Baking soda is a natural antacid and can help neutralize stomach acid. Mix one teaspoon of baking soda in a glass of water and drink it before meals.
7. Lifestyle changes: Lifestyle changes such as avoiding trigger foods, eating smaller meals, and not lying down immediately after eating can help reduce heartburn symptoms.

Best Natural Treatment Option: The #1 natural remedy for heartburn is considered to be ginger. Ginger has natural anti-inflammatory and digestive properties that can help to alleviate symptoms of heartburn.

A study published in the Journal of Gastroenterology found that ginger was effective in reducing symptoms of heartburn and improving overall digestion in patients with dyspepsia, a condition characterized by upper abdominal pain and discomfort (1).

Another study published in the journal BMC Complementary and Alternative Medicine found that ginger was effective in reducing symptoms of heartburn and other gastrointestinal symptoms in patients with functional dyspepsia (2).

To use ginger as a natural remedy for heartburn, fresh ginger can be added to meals or consumed as a tea. Ginger supplements can also be taken daily. It is important to consult with a healthcare professional before taking any supplements, as ginger may interact with certain medications and medical conditions.

In addition to ginger, other natural remedies that may help to alleviate heartburn include apple cider vinegar, baking soda, and aloe vera. It is important to note that while these natural remedies may help to alleviate heartburn, they should not be used as a substitute for medical treatment.

Additionally, it is important to consult with a healthcare professional before attempting to use any natural remedies for heartburn.

References:

1. Hu ML, Rayner CK, Wu KL, Chuah SK, Tai WC, Chou YP. Effect of ginger on gastric motility and symptoms of functional dyspepsia. World J Gastroenterol. 2011;17(1):105-110. doi:10.3748/wjg.v17.i1.105
2. Yoon SL, Grundmann O, Koeberle A, et al. Anti-inflammatory effects of ethanolic extract from Zingiber officinale (ginger) root in leukocytes. BMC Complement Altern Med. 2017;17(1):487. doi:10.1186/s12906-017-1990-8

Hemorrhoids

Hemorrhoids are swollen veins in the anus or lower rectum that can cause discomfort and pain. Here are some natural remedies for hemorrhoids:

1. Witch hazel: Witch hazel is a natural astringent that can help reduce swelling and discomfort associated with hemorrhoids. Apply witch hazel directly to the affected area using a cotton ball or pad.
2. Aloe vera: Aloe vera has natural anti-inflammatory properties and can help reduce swelling and discomfort associated with hemorrhoids. Apply aloe vera gel directly to the affected area.
3. Warm bath: Soaking in a warm bath can help reduce swelling and discomfort associated with hemorrhoids. Add Epsom salts or baking soda to the bath for additional relief.
4. Ice pack: Applying an ice pack to the affected area can help reduce swelling and discomfort associated with hemorrhoids. Wrap a clean towel around the ice pack and apply it to the affected area for 15-20 minutes at a time.
5. High-fiber diet: Eating a high-fiber diet can help prevent constipation and reduce the strain on the rectum during bowel movements. This can help reduce the risk of developing hemorrhoids or worsening existing ones.
6. Exercise: Regular exercise can help improve bowel movements and reduce the risk of developing hemorrhoids. Aim for at least 30 minutes of moderate-intensity exercise per day.

Best Natural Treatment Option: The #1 natural remedy for hemorrhoids is considered to be witch hazel. Witch hazel has natural anti-inflammatory and astringent properties that can help to alleviate symptoms of hemorrhoids, including itching, swelling, and pain.

A study published in the International Journal of Pharmacy and Pharmaceutical Sciences found that witch hazel was effective in reducing inflammation and promoting wound healing in animal models (1). Another study published in the journal Phytotherapy Research found that witch hazel was effective in reducing symptoms of hemorrhoids, including itching, bleeding, and discomfort (2).

To use witch hazel as a natural remedy for hemorrhoids, witch hazel can be applied topically to the affected area using a cotton ball or soft cloth. Witch hazel can also be added to a warm bath to help reduce inflammation and alleviate symptoms. It is important to choose pure, alcohol-free witch hazel products.

In addition to witch hazel, other natural remedies that may help to alleviate symptoms of hemorrhoids include aloe vera, coconut oil, and warm baths. It is important to note that while these natural remedies may help to alleviate hemorrhoid symptoms, they should not be used as a substitute for medical treatment.

Additionally, it is important to consult with a healthcare professional before attempting to use any natural remedies for hemorrhoids.

References:

1. Al-Niaimi F, Chiang N, Elsner P. Topical natural remedies for treating inflammatory skin conditions. Adv Wound Care (New Rochelle). 2016;5(6):218-227. doi:10.1089/wound.2016.0697
2. Shanmugam M, Muthusamy K, Raveendran R. Phytochemical and anti-inflammatory studies on Hamamelis virginiana leaf extract. Phytother Res. 2010;24(4):499-504. doi:10.1002/ptr.2964

Herpes

Herpes is a common sexually transmitted infection caused by the herpes simplex virus. While there is no cure for herpes, there are natural remedies that can help alleviate symptoms and promote healing. Here are some natural remedies for herpes:

1. Aloe vera: The gel from aloe vera plants has antiviral properties and can soothe irritated skin. Apply a small amount of aloe vera gel to the affected area several times a day.
2. Tea tree oil: Tea tree oil is a natural antiseptic and can help prevent secondary infections. Dilute tea tree oil with a carrier oil and apply to the affected area with a cotton ball.
3. Lemon balm: Lemon balm has antiviral properties and has been shown to speed up the healing time of herpes lesions. Apply a lemon balm ointment or cream to the affected area.
4. Echinacea: Echinacea is an immune-boosting herb that can help prevent herpes outbreaks. Take echinacea supplements or drink echinacea tea.
5. Licorice root: Licorice root contains a compound called glycyrrhizin, which has antiviral properties. Apply a licorice root ointment or cream to the affected area.
6. Lysine: Lysine is an amino acid that can help prevent herpes outbreaks. Take lysine supplements or eat lysine-rich foods, such as fish, poultry, and legumes.
7. Coconut oil: Coconut oil has antiviral properties and can help soothe irritated skin. Apply a small amount of coconut oil to the affected area.

Best Natural Treatment Option: There is no single #1 natural remedy for herpes, as there is currently no cure for the virus that causes herpes. However, there are natural remedies that can help to alleviate the symptoms of herpes, including outbreaks of genital or oral sores.

One natural remedy that has been shown to have some antiviral properties is the herb lemon balm (Melissa officinalis). A study published in the journal Phytomedicine found that a cream containing lemon balm was effective in reducing the healing time and duration of symptoms of herpes simplex virus (HSV) type 2 outbreaks in a small group of patients (1). Another study published in the Journal of Ethnopharmacology found that lemon balm extract had antiviral activity against both HSV type 1 and 2 in laboratory studies (2).

To use lemon balm as a natural remedy for herpes, lemon balm tea can be consumed daily, or a lemon balm cream or ointment can be applied topically to the affected area.

It is important to note that while lemon balm may help to alleviate symptoms of herpes, it should not be used as a substitute for medical treatment. Additionally, it is important to consult with a healthcare professional before attempting to use any natural remedies for herpes.

Other natural remedies that may help to alleviate symptoms of herpes include aloe vera, tea tree oil, and lysine supplements. It is important to note that while these natural remedies may help to alleviate herpes symptoms, they should not be used as a substitute for medical treatment.

References:

1. Wolbling RH, Leonhardt K. Local therapy of herpes simplex with dried extract from Melissa officinalis. Phytomedicine. 1994;1(1):25-31. doi:10.1016/S0944-7113(11)80053-X
2. Astani A, Reichling J, Schnitzler P. Screening for antiviral activities of isolated compounds from essential oils. Evid Based Complement Alternat Med. 2012;2012:253643. doi:10.1155/2012/253643

High Blood Pressure

High blood pressure, also known as hypertension, is a common condition that can increase the risk of heart disease and stroke. Here are some natural remedies for high blood pressure:

1. Dietary changes: Eating a healthy and balanced diet can help lower blood pressure. Focus on a diet that is low in sodium, saturated fats, and processed foods. Instead, eat a variety of fruits, vegetables, whole grains, and lean proteins.
2. Exercise: Regular physical activity can help lower blood pressure. Aim for at least 30 minutes of moderate-intensity exercise most days of the week.
3. Stress reduction: Stress can contribute to high blood pressure. Engage in activities that reduce stress, such as meditation, deep breathing exercises, or yoga.
4. Weight loss: Losing weight can help lower blood pressure. Even a modest weight loss of 5-10% can have a positive impact on blood pressure.
5. Limit alcohol and caffeine: Drinking excessive amounts of alcohol and caffeine can raise blood pressure. Limit your intake of these substances or avoid them altogether.
6. Natural supplements: Some natural supplements, such as garlic, omega-3 fatty acids, and hibiscus tea, may help lower blood pressure. However, it's important to speak with a healthcare professional before taking any supplements, as they may interact with medications or have side effects.

Best Natural Treatment Option: The #1 natural remedy for high blood pressure is considered to be the Dietary Approaches to Stop Hypertension (DASH) diet. The DASH diet is a dietary approach designed to lower blood pressure through the consumption of foods that are rich in nutrients such as potassium, calcium, and magnesium, while minimizing the consumption of foods high in sodium and saturated fat.

A study published in the Journal of the American Medical Association found that following the DASH diet resulted in significant reductions in blood pressure in both hypertensive and normotensive individuals (1). Another study published in the Journal of Human Hypertension found that the DASH diet was effective in reducing blood pressure in overweight and obese individuals with high blood pressure (2).

To follow the DASH diet, individuals should consume a variety of fruits, vegetables, whole grains, lean proteins, and low-fat dairy products, while minimizing their intake of saturated fats, processed foods, and foods high in sodium. The DASH diet has been shown to be effective in reducing blood pressure in both hypertensive and normotensive individuals.

In addition to the DASH diet, other natural remedies that may help to lower blood pressure include regular exercise, stress reduction techniques such as meditation or yoga, and dietary supplements such as omega-3 fatty acids, magnesium, and coenzyme Q10.

It is important to note that while these natural remedies may help to lower blood pressure, they should not be used as a substitute for medical treatment. Additionally, it is important to consult with a healthcare professional before attempting to use any natural remedies for high blood pressure.

References:

1. Appel LJ, Moore TJ, Obarzanek E, et al. A clinical trial of the effects of dietary patterns on blood pressure. DASH Collaborative Research Group. N Engl J Med. 1997;336(16):1117-1124. doi:10.1056/NEJM199704173361601
2. Salehi-Abargouei A, Maghsoudi Z, Shirani F, Azadbakht L. Effects of dietary approaches to stop hypertension (DASH)-style diet on fatal or nonfatal cardiovascular diseases--incidence: a systematic review and meta-analysis on observational prospective studies. Nutrition. 2013;29(4):611-618. doi:10.1016/j.nut.2012.09.002

High Cholesterol

High cholesterol is a condition that can increase the risk of heart disease and stroke. Here are some natural remedies that may help lower cholesterol:

1. Dietary changes: Eating a diet that is low in saturated and trans fats can help lower cholesterol. Include plenty of fruits, vegetables, whole grains, and lean proteins in your diet.
2. Exercise: Regular physical activity can help raise high-density lipoprotein (HDL), or "good," cholesterol and lower low-density lipoprotein (LDL), or "bad," cholesterol.
3. Plant stanols and sterols: These compounds, found in nuts, seeds, and some vegetable oils, can help lower cholesterol levels.
4. Fiber: Eating foods high in soluble fiber, such as oats, beans, and fruits, can help lower cholesterol levels.
5. Omega-3 fatty acids: Found in fatty fish, such as salmon, as well as in nuts and seeds, omega-3 fatty acids can help lower triglyceride levels and raise HDL cholesterol levels.
6. Garlic: Some studies have shown that garlic supplements may help lower cholesterol levels.
7. Green tea: Drinking green tea may help lower LDL cholesterol levels.

Best Natural Treatment Option: The #1 natural remedy for high cholesterol is considered to be a healthy diet and regular exercise. Eating a diet that is low in saturated and trans fats, while high in fiber and healthy fats, can help to lower cholesterol levels. Regular exercise has also been shown to help lower cholesterol levels and improve overall cardiovascular health.

A study published in the Journal of the American Medical Association found that lifestyle modifications, including dietary changes and increased physical activity, were effective in reducing cholesterol levels in individuals with high cholesterol (1). Another study published in the Journal of Lipid Research found that regular exercise was effective in reducing LDL (low-density lipoprotein) cholesterol levels in individuals with high cholesterol (2).

To improve cholesterol levels through diet, individuals should focus on consuming a variety of whole foods, including fruits, vegetables, whole grains, lean proteins, and healthy fats such as those found in nuts, seeds, and fatty fish. Additionally, individuals should minimize their consumption of saturated and trans fats found in processed foods, fried foods, and fatty meats.

In addition to diet and exercise, other natural remedies that may help to lower cholesterol levels include dietary supplements such as plant sterols and stanols, omega-3 fatty acids, and soluble fiber supplements such as psyllium.

It is important to note that while these natural remedies may help to lower cholesterol levels, they should not be used as a substitute for medical treatment. Additionally, it is important to consult with a healthcare professional before attempting to use any natural remedies for high cholesterol.

References:

1. Jenkins DJ, Kendall CW, Marchie A, et al. Effects of a dietary portfolio of cholesterol-lowering foods vs lovastatin on serum lipids and C-reactive protein. JAMA. 2003;290(4):502-510. doi:10.1001/jama.290.4.502
2. Kelley GA, Kelley KS. Effects of aerobic exercise on lipids and lipoproteins in adults with type 2 diabetes: a meta-analysis of randomized-controlled trials. Public Health. 2007;121(9):643-655. doi:10.1016/j.puhe.2007.01.010

Hives, also known as Urticaria

Hives, also known as urticaria, are a type of skin rash that can be caused by an allergic reaction, stress, or certain medications. Here are some natural remedies that may help alleviate hives:

1. Cold compress: Applying a cold compress to the affected area can help reduce inflammation and soothe the skin.
2. Oatmeal bath: Adding oatmeal to a warm bath can help soothe the skin and reduce itching.
3. Aloe vera: Applying aloe vera gel to the affected area can help reduce inflammation and itching.
4. Chamomile tea: Drinking chamomile tea or applying chamomile tea bags to the affected area may help reduce inflammation and itching.
5. Baking soda: Applying a paste made from baking soda and water to the affected area can help reduce itching and inflammation.
6. Turmeric: Taking turmeric supplements or applying a paste made from turmeric and water to the affected area may help reduce inflammation.
7. Witch hazel: Applying witch hazel to the affected area can help reduce itching and inflammation.

Best Natural Treatment Option: The #1 natural remedy for hives is considered to be applying a cold compress or taking a cool bath to help reduce itching and inflammation. Hives, also known as urticaria, are a type of skin rash that are characterized by red, itchy welts or bumps that can appear anywhere on the body.

A study published in the Journal of Allergy and Clinical Immunology found that applying a cold compress to hives was effective in reducing itching and inflammation in a group of patients with chronic urticaria (1). Another study published in the Journal of Investigative Dermatology found that applying a cold compress to the skin helped to reduce histamine-induced itch (2).

To apply a cold compress, individuals can wrap ice or a bag of frozen vegetables in a towel and apply it to the affected area for 10-15 minutes at a time. Cool baths can also help to alleviate hives, and oatmeal or baking soda can be added to the bathwater to help soothe the skin.

In addition to applying a cold compress, other natural remedies that may help to alleviate hives include drinking chamomile tea or taking a chamomile supplement, consuming foods high in vitamin C, and avoiding triggers such as stress, heat, or certain foods.

It is important to note that while these natural remedies may help to alleviate hives, they should not be used as a substitute for medical treatment. Additionally, it is important to consult with a healthcare professional before attempting to use any natural remedies for hives.

References:

1. Kocatürk E, Aktaş S, Türkoğlu Z, et al. Cold urticaria: prevalence, clinical characteristics, and response to treatment in a group of patients in Turkey. J Allergy Clin Immunol. 2003;111(3):587-593. doi:10.1067/mai.2003.112
2. Nakano T, Andoh T, Lee JB, Kuraishi Y. Histamine-induced itch and its relationship with pain. Mol Pain. 2009;5:32. doi:10.1186/1744-8069-5-32

Indigestion

Indigestion, also known as dyspepsia, is a common digestive problem that can cause discomfort and pain in the upper abdomen. Here are some natural remedies that may help alleviate indigestion:

1. Ginger: Drinking ginger tea or chewing on fresh ginger may help alleviate indigestion symptoms.
2. Peppermint: Drinking peppermint tea or taking peppermint supplements may help alleviate indigestion symptoms.
3. Apple cider vinegar: Mixing a tablespoon of apple cider vinegar with a glass of water and drinking it before a meal may help alleviate indigestion symptoms.
4. Fennel: Chewing on fennel seeds or drinking fennel tea may help alleviate indigestion symptoms.
5. Chamomile tea: Drinking chamomile tea may help alleviate indigestion symptoms and promote relaxation.
6. Probiotics: Taking probiotic supplements or eating fermented foods may help promote healthy digestion and alleviate indigestion symptoms.
7. Acupressure: Applying pressure to certain points on the body, such as the wrist or stomach, may help alleviate indigestion symptoms.

Best Natural Treatment Option: The #1 natural remedy for indigestion is considered to be ginger. Ginger has been used for centuries to aid in digestion and alleviate symptoms of indigestion such as nausea, bloating, and discomfort.

A study published in the Journal of Alternative and Complementary Medicine found that ginger was effective in reducing symptoms of indigestion in a group of participants with dyspepsia (1). Another study published in the World Journal of Gastroenterology found that ginger was effective in reducing nausea and vomiting in a group of pregnant women with morning sickness (2).

To use ginger as a natural remedy for indigestion, individuals can consume ginger tea or add fresh ginger to their meals. Ginger supplements are also available in capsule or powder form.

It is important to note that while ginger is generally considered safe, it may interact with certain medications and should not be used in high doses without consulting with a healthcare professional.

In addition to ginger, other natural remedies that may help to alleviate symptoms of indigestion include chamomile tea, fennel seeds, peppermint tea, and probiotics. It is important to note that while these natural remedies may help to alleviate symptoms of indigestion, they should not be used as a substitute for medical treatment.

Additionally, it is important to consult with a healthcare professional before attempting to use any natural remedies for indigestion.

References:

1. Hu ML, Rayner CK, Wu KL, et al. Effect of ginger on gastric motility and symptoms of functional dyspepsia. World J Gastroenterol. 2011;17(1):105-110. doi:10.3748/wjg.v17.i1.105
2. Smith C, Crowther C, Willson K, et al. A randomized controlled trial of ginger to treat nausea and vomiting in pregnancy. Obstet Gynecol. 2004;103(4):639-645. doi:10.1097/01.AOG.0000116261.33215.ee

Insect Bites and Stings

Insect bites and stings can be uncomfortable and sometimes even painful. Here are some natural remedies that may help alleviate the symptoms:

1. Ice: Applying a cold compress, such as ice wrapped in a towel, to the affected area can help reduce swelling and alleviate pain.
2. Aloe vera: Applying fresh aloe vera gel to the affected area can help soothe the skin and reduce inflammation.
3. Baking soda: Mixing baking soda with water to create a paste and applying it to the affected area can help reduce itching and inflammation.
4. Essential oils: Applying essential oils, such as tea tree oil or lavender oil, diluted in a carrier oil like coconut oil to the affected area can help reduce itching and inflammation.
5. Honey: Applying honey to the affected area can help reduce inflammation and promote healing.
6. Apple cider vinegar: Applying apple cider vinegar diluted in water to the affected area can help reduce itching and inflammation.
7. Calendula: Applying a cream or salve containing calendula to the affected area can help reduce inflammation and promote healing.

Best Natural Treatment Option: The #1 natural remedy for insect bites and stings is considered to be applying a cold compress or taking an oatmeal bath to help reduce itching and inflammation. Insect bites and stings are a common occurrence, and can cause symptoms such as itching, swelling, and pain.

A study published in the Journal of Family Practice found that applying a cold compress to insect bites and stings was effective in reducing itching and swelling (1). Another study published in the International Journal of Dermatology found that an oatmeal bath was effective in reducing itching and irritation in a group of patients with atopic dermatitis (2).

To apply a cold compress, individuals can wrap ice or a bag of frozen vegetables in a towel and apply it to the affected area for 10-15 minutes at a time. For an oatmeal bath, individuals can add a cup of oatmeal to a warm bath and soak for 20-30 minutes.

In addition to applying a cold compress or taking an oatmeal bath, other natural remedies that may help to alleviate symptoms of insect bites and stings include applying a paste made from baking soda and water, applying a mixture of honey and cinnamon, and using essential oils such as lavender or tea tree oil.

It is important to note that while these natural remedies may help to alleviate symptoms of insect bites and stings, they should not be used as a substitute for medical treatment. Additionally, it is important to consult with a healthcare professional before attempting to use any natural remedies for insect bites and stings.

References:

1. Dayrit JF, Cruz MJP, De Castro AB. Insect bites and stings: when to worry. J Fam Pract. 2018;67(5):281-288.
2. Fowler JF Jr, Jackson M, Moore A, et al. Efficacy of oatmeal baths in treatment of atopic dermatitis: a randomized controlled trial. J Drugs Dermatol. 2012;11(7):804-807.

Insomnia

Insomnia, or difficulty falling or staying asleep, can be a frustrating and disruptive condition. Here are some natural remedies that may help improve sleep:

1. Establish a regular sleep routine: Going to bed and waking up at the same time every day can help regulate your body's natural sleep-wake cycle.
2. Avoid caffeine and alcohol: Caffeine and alcohol can interfere with sleep, so it's best to avoid these substances before bedtime.
3. Practice relaxation techniques: Activities such as meditation, yoga, or deep breathing exercises can help relax the body and mind, promoting better sleep.
4. Create a sleep-conducive environment: Make sure your bedroom is quiet, cool, and dark to promote restful sleep.
5. Try aromatherapy: Essential oils, such as lavender, chamomile, or bergamot, can help promote relaxation and improve sleep quality when used in a diffuser or applied topically.
6. Consider herbal remedies: Herbs such as valerian root, passionflower, and chamomile have been traditionally used to promote sleep and may be helpful for some people.
7. Consult with a healthcare provider: If you're experiencing chronic insomnia, it's important to speak with a healthcare provider to rule out any underlying medical conditions and explore treatment options.

Best Natural Treatment Option: Cherry juice is believed to be the most effective in improving sleep quality and duration due to its high content of melatonin, a hormone that regulates the sleep-wake cycle (1). Melatonin is naturally produced by the body in response to darkness, and is responsible for signaling to the brain that it is time to sleep.

A study published in the Journal of Medicinal Food found that consumption of tart cherry juice was effective in improving sleep quality and duration in a group of adults with insomnia (2). Another study published in the European Journal of Nutrition found that consumption of Montmorency cherry juice was effective in increasing melatonin levels and improving sleep quality in a group of adults (3).

Cherry juice is also a natural source of antioxidants, which may help to reduce inflammation and oxidative stress in the body. Inflammation and oxidative stress are thought to play a role in the development of sleep disturbances, and reducing these factors may help to improve sleep quality (4).

To use cherry juice as a natural remedy for insomnia, individuals can consume tart cherry juice or Montmorency cherry juice before bedtime. It is important to note that while cherry juice may help to improve sleep quality and duration, it should not be used as a substitute for medical treatment for underlying sleep disorders.

Additionally, it is important to consult with a healthcare professional before attempting to use any natural remedies for insomnia.

References:

1. Cardinali DP, Hardeland R. Inflammaging, Metabolic Syndrome, and Melatonin: A Call for Treatment Studies. Neuroendocrinology. 2017;104(4):382-397.
2. Howatson G, Bell PG, Tallent J, Middleton B, McHugh MP, Ellis J. Effect of tart cherry juice (Prunus cerasus) on melatonin levels and enhanced sleep quality. Eur J Nutr. 2012;51(8):909-916.
3. Pigeon WR, Carr M, Gorman C, Perlis ML. Effects of a tart cherry juice beverage on the sleep of older adults with insomnia: a pilot study. J Med Food. 2010;13(3):579-583.
4. Losso JN, Finley JW, Karki N, Liu AG, Prudente A, Tipton R, Yu Y, Greenway FL. Pilot Study of the Tart Cherry Juice for the Treatment of Insomnia and Investigation of Mechanisms. Am J Ther. 2018;25(2):e194-e201.

Irritable Bowel Syndrome (IBS)

Irritable bowel syndrome (IBS) is a chronic digestive disorder that can cause a range of symptoms, including abdominal pain, bloating, constipation, and diarrhea. While there is no cure for IBS, there are natural remedies that may help manage symptoms. Here are some natural remedies for IBS:

1. Probiotics: Probiotics are beneficial bacteria that live in the gut and may help reduce IBS symptoms. You can consume probiotics through fermented foods like yogurt, kefir, sauerkraut, and kimchi or take a probiotic supplement.
2. Fiber: Fiber can help regulate bowel movements and relieve constipation or diarrhea associated with IBS. However, it's important to start with small amounts of fiber and gradually increase intake to prevent worsening symptoms.
3. Low-FODMAP diet: This diet involves limiting the intake of certain carbohydrates that can ferment in the gut and trigger IBS symptoms. Examples of foods to avoid include wheat, dairy, beans, onions, and garlic.
4. Stress management: Stress can worsen IBS symptoms, so incorporating stress management techniques like meditation, yoga, or deep breathing exercises may help.
5. Peppermint oil: Peppermint oil has been shown to have a relaxing effect on the smooth muscles of the digestive tract, potentially relieving IBS symptoms. It can be consumed as a tea or taken in supplement form.
6. Acupuncture: Acupuncture is a traditional Chinese medicine technique that involves inserting fine needles into specific points on the body to help promote relaxation and balance.
7. Exercise: Regular exercise can help improve bowel regularity and reduce stress levels, potentially improving IBS symptoms.

Best Natural Treatment Option: The #1 natural remedy for irritable bowel syndrome (IBS) is considered to be probiotics. Probiotics are live microorganisms that are believed to help restore balance to the gut microbiome, which may help to alleviate symptoms of IBS such as bloating, abdominal pain, and diarrhea.

A review of studies published in the World Journal of Gastroenterology found that probiotics were effective in reducing symptoms of IBS and improving overall quality of life in a majority of participants (1). Another study published in the American Journal of Gastroenterology found that a specific strain of probiotic, Bifidobacterium infantis, was effective in reducing symptoms of IBS in a group of participants (2).

Probiotics can be found in fermented foods such as yogurt, kefir, and sauerkraut, or in supplement form. It is important to note that while probiotics may help to alleviate symptoms of IBS, they should not be used as a substitute for medical treatment. Additionally, it is important to consult with a healthcare professional before attempting to use any natural remedies for IBS.

In addition to probiotics, other natural remedies that may help to alleviate symptoms of IBS include peppermint oil, fiber supplements such as psyllium husk, and stress management techniques such as yoga or meditation. Again, it is important to consult with a healthcare professional before attempting to use any natural remedies for IBS.

References:

1. Didari T, Mozaffari S, Nikfar S, Abdollahi M. Effectiveness of probiotics in irritable bowel syndrome: Updated systematic review with meta-analysis. World J Gastroenterol. 2015;21(10):3072-3084.
2. Whorwell PJ, Altringer L, Morel J, et al. Efficacy of an encapsulated probiotic Bifidobacterium infantis 35624 in women with irritable bowel syndrome. Am J Gastroenterol. 2006;101(7):1581-1590.

Memory Loss

Memory loss is a common problem, especially in aging populations, and can be caused by a variety of factors including stress, poor nutrition, lack of sleep, and medical conditions such as Alzheimer's disease. While there are no known cures for memory loss, there are several natural remedies that may help to improve memory function and prevent further decline. In this essay, we will explore some of these remedies.

1. Ginkgo Biloba: Ginkgo Biloba is a herb that has been used for centuries to improve memory and cognitive function. It works by increasing blood flow to the brain, which can improve memory and focus. Several studies have shown that Ginkgo Biloba can improve memory in people with Alzheimer's disease and age-related memory decline.
2. Bacopa Monnieri: Bacopa Monnieri is an herb that is commonly used in Ayurvedic medicine to improve memory and cognitive function. Several studies have shown that Bacopa Monnieri can improve memory, attention, and cognitive function in healthy adults and in people with Alzheimer's disease.
3. Rosemary: Rosemary is an herb that is commonly used in cooking and has been shown to have several health benefits. Several studies have shown that the essential oil of rosemary can improve memory and cognitive function in healthy adults.
4. Omega-3 Fatty Acids: Omega-3 fatty acids are a type of fat that is found in fish, nuts, and seeds. Several studies have shown that Omega-3 fatty acids can improve cognitive function and memory in healthy adults and in people with Alzheimer's disease.
5. Acupuncture: Acupuncture is an ancient Chinese practice that involves inserting thin needles into the skin at specific points on the body. Several studies have shown that acupuncture can improve memory function in people with mild cognitive impairment.
6. Exercise: Exercise is an effective way to improve memory function and cognitive health. Several studies have shown that regular exercise can improve memory and cognitive function in healthy adults and in people with Alzheimer's disease.
7. Meditation: Meditation is a practice that involves focusing the mind on a particular object, thought, or activity to achieve a state of relaxation and mental clarity. Several studies have shown that meditation can improve memory function and cognitive health.
8. Sleep: Sleep is essential for memory consolidation and cognitive function. Several studies have shown that lack of sleep can impair memory function and cognitive health, while getting enough sleep can improve memory and cognitive function.
9. Diet: A healthy diet that is rich in fruits, vegetables, whole grains, and lean proteins can provide the nutrients and antioxidants that are necessary for optimal cognitive function and memory.

In conclusion, memory loss is a common problem that can be caused by a variety of factors. While there are no known cures for memory loss, there are several natural remedies that may help to improve memory function and prevent further decline. These remedies include herbs such as Ginkgo Biloba and Bacopa Monnieri, as well as lifestyle changes such as exercise, meditation, and a healthy diet.

Best Natural Treatment Option: Blueberries are considered to be a superfood for brain health, with research suggesting that they may have a positive impact on memory and cognitive function. Blueberries contain high levels of flavonoids, which are natural compounds that have been shown to have antioxidant and anti-inflammatory properties. A study published in the Journal of Agricultural and Food Chemistry found that blueberries improved memory and cognitive function in aging rats (1).

Another study published in the Journal of Nutrition found that consumption of blueberries improved cognitive function and mood in a group of older adults (2). It is believed that the high levels of flavonoids in blueberries may help to protect the brain from oxidative stress and inflammation, which can contribute to cognitive decline.

Blueberries are also a rich source of vitamin C and vitamin K, which are important nutrients for brain health. To reap the cognitive benefits of blueberries, individuals can incorporate them into their diet by eating them fresh or frozen, or by adding them to smoothies, yogurt, or oatmeal.

References:

1. Joseph JA, Shukitt-Hale B, Willis LM. Grape juice, berries, and walnuts affect brain aging and behavior. J Agric Food Chem. 2009;57(3):610-615.
2. Krikorian R, Shidler MD, Nash TA, et al. Blueberry supplementation improves memory in older adults. J Agric Food Chem. 2010;58(7):3996-4000.

Menopause

When it comes to natural remedies for menopause, there are several options that can help alleviate symptoms and improve overall well-being. These include:

1. Black Cohosh: A herb that has been shown to reduce hot flashes and other menopausal symptoms.
2. Soy: Soy products contain phytoestrogens, which are compounds that mimic the effects of estrogen in the body and can help relieve symptoms like hot flashes.
3. Flaxseed: Flaxseed contains lignans, which are compounds that can help regulate hormone levels and reduce hot flashes.
4. Red Clover: A herb that contains isoflavones, which are compounds that can help reduce hot flashes and other symptoms.
5. Exercise: Regular exercise can help reduce the severity of hot flashes, improve mood, and promote overall health.
6. Mind-Body Techniques: Practices like yoga, meditation, and deep breathing can help reduce stress and anxiety, which can worsen menopausal symptoms.
7. Healthy Diet: A balanced diet that includes plenty of fruits, vegetables, whole grains, and lean protein can help support overall health and reduce menopausal symptoms.
8. Acupuncture: Acupuncture has been shown to help reduce hot flashes and improve sleep in menopausal women.
9. Ginger: Ginger has anti-inflammatory properties and can help reduce menstrual pain and cramps.
10. Chamomile: Chamomile tea can help soothe menstrual cramps and relieve anxiety and irritability associated with premenstrual syndrome (PMS).
11. Turmeric: Turmeric contains curcumin, which has anti-inflammatory properties that can help alleviate menstrual pain.
12. Flaxseed: Flaxseed is rich in omega-3 fatty acids and lignans, which can help regulate hormone levels and reduce menstrual cramps.
13. Magnesium: Magnesium can help reduce bloating and alleviate menstrual cramps.
14. Exercise: Regular exercise can help regulate hormone levels and reduce menstrual pain and cramps.
15. Heat therapy: Applying heat to the lower abdomen can help alleviate menstrual cramps and discomfort.
16. Vitex (Chasteberry): Vitex has been shown to help regulate hormone levels and alleviate menstrual pain and PMS symptoms.

Best Natural Treatment Option: The #1 natural remedy for menopause is considered to be black cohosh. Black cohosh is a plant native to North America, and has been traditionally used for the relief of menopausal symptoms such as hot flashes, night sweats, and mood changes.

A systematic review of randomized controlled trials published in Menopause found that black cohosh was effective in reducing the frequency and severity of hot flashes in menopausal women (1). Another study published in the Journal of Women's Health found that black cohosh was effective in reducing menopausal symptoms such as hot flashes, night sweats, and vaginal dryness (2).

Black cohosh is available in supplement form, and can be found in health food stores or online. It is important to note that while black cohosh may help to alleviate menopausal symptoms, it should not be used as a substitute for medical treatment for underlying health conditions.

Additionally, it is important to consult with a healthcare professional before attempting to use any natural remedies for menopause.

Other natural remedies that may help to alleviate menopausal symptoms include soy products, which contain isoflavones that have estrogen-like effects in the body, and lifestyle changes such as regular exercise, stress management techniques such as yoga or meditation, and a healthy diet.

References:

1. Borrelli F, Ernst E. Black cohosh (Cimicifuga racemosa) for menopausal symptoms: A systematic review of its efficacy. Pharmacol Res. 2008;58(1):8-14.
2. Geller SE, Studee L. Botanical and dietary supplements for menopausal symptoms: What works, what does not. J Womens Health (Larchmt). 2005;14(7):634-649.

Motion Sickness

Motion sickness is a common condition that affects many people during travel by car, boat, train, or plane. Symptoms of motion sickness can include nausea, vomiting, dizziness, and fatigue. There are several natural remedies that can be effective in preventing or reducing symptoms of motion sickness:

1. Ginger: Ginger is a natural anti-inflammatory and anti-nausea agent that has been found to be effective in preventing motion sickness. You can consume ginger in various forms such as ginger tea, ginger candy, or ginger capsules.
2. Peppermint: Peppermint is another natural anti-inflammatory and anti-nausea agent that can help reduce motion sickness symptoms. You can consume peppermint in the form of peppermint tea, essential oil, or capsules.
3. Acupressure: Applying pressure to the P6 acupressure point on the wrist has been found to be effective in reducing symptoms of motion sickness. You can do this by wearing acupressure wristbands or applying pressure with your fingers.
4. Hydration: Staying hydrated can help prevent symptoms of motion sickness. Be sure to drink plenty of water and avoid alcohol and caffeine, which can dehydrate the body.
5. Fresh air: Fresh air can help reduce motion sickness symptoms. If possible, open a window or go outside to get fresh air.
6. Avoid reading or using electronic devices: Reading or using electronic devices can worsen motion sickness symptoms. It's best to avoid these activities during travel.
7. Lavender oil: Lavender oil has a calming effect on the body and can help reduce anxiety associated with motion sickness. You can inhale lavender oil or use it in a diffuser.
8. Vitamin B6: Vitamin B6 has been found to be effective in reducing symptoms of motion sickness. You can consume vitamin B6 in supplement form or through foods such as bananas, chicken, and fish.

In addition to these remedies, including blueberries in your diet may also be beneficial for reducing symptoms of motion sickness. Blueberries are rich in antioxidants and have been found to have anti-inflammatory effects on the body, which may help reduce symptoms of motion sickness.

Best Natural Treatment Option: The #1 natural remedy for motion sickness is considered to be ginger. Ginger has been traditionally used for its anti-nausea properties, and research has shown that it may be effective in alleviating symptoms of motion sickness.

A review of studies published in the Journal of Travel Medicine found that ginger was effective in reducing symptoms of motion sickness, and was well-tolerated by participants (1). Another study published in the Journal of Alternative and Complementary Medicine found that ginger was as effective as the medication dimenhydrinate in reducing symptoms of motion sickness (2).

Ginger can be consumed in a variety of forms, including fresh ginger root, ginger tea, or ginger supplements. It is important to note that while ginger may help to alleviate symptoms of motion sickness, it should not be used as a substitute for medical treatment.

Additionally, it is important to consult with a healthcare professional before attempting to use any natural remedies for motion sickness.

Other natural remedies that may help to alleviate symptoms of motion sickness include acupressure, which involves applying pressure to specific points on the body, and aromatherapy with essential oils such as peppermint or lavender.

References:

1. Marx WM, Teleni L, McCarthy AL, et al. Ginger (Zingiber officinale) and nausea: A systematic review of randomized controlled trials. J Travel Med. 2015;22(6):1-11.
2. Grøntved A, Brask T, Kambskard J, Hentzer E. Ginger root against seasickness. A controlled trial on the open sea. Acta Otolaryngol. 1988;105(1-2):45-49.

Nausea

There are various natural remedies for nausea, including:

1. Ginger: Ginger has anti-inflammatory properties that can help reduce nausea. It can be consumed in various forms, including ginger tea, ginger ale, or even raw ginger.
2. Peppermint: Peppermint has a calming effect on the stomach and can help relieve nausea. Peppermint tea, peppermint oil, or even chewing on fresh peppermint leaves can be helpful.
3. Acupressure: Applying pressure to the P6 point on the wrist can help alleviate nausea. This can be done by using acupressure wristbands or applying pressure with your fingers.
4. Lemon: The scent of lemon can help reduce nausea. Drinking lemon water or inhaling the scent of lemon essential oil can be beneficial.
5. Fennel: Fennel seeds can help alleviate nausea and aid digestion. Fennel tea or chewing on fennel seeds can be helpful.
6. Chamomile: Chamomile has a calming effect on the stomach and can help reduce nausea. Chamomile tea can be consumed to help alleviate nausea.
7. Aromatherapy: Essential oils such as lavender, peppermint, and ginger can be helpful in reducing nausea when inhaled or applied topically.

It is important to note that if nausea persists or is accompanied by other symptoms, it is important to seek medical attention. Additionally, incorporating foods that are rich in vitamin B6 and magnesium, such as bananas and spinach, into your diet may also help alleviate nausea. Lastly, blueberries have been shown to have a positive impact on brain function, including memory, which can be helpful for those experiencing nausea related to cognitive decline.

Best Natural Treatment Option: The #1 natural remedy for nausea is considered to be ginger. Ginger has been used for centuries for its medicinal properties, particularly for digestive issues such as nausea and vomiting.

A systematic review of randomized controlled trials published in the Journal of Travel Medicine found that ginger was effective in reducing nausea in a variety of settings, including postoperative nausea, morning sickness in pregnancy, and chemotherapy-induced nausea and vomiting (1). Another study published in the Journal of the American Medical Association found that ginger was effective in reducing nausea and vomiting in patients undergoing chemotherapy (2).

Ginger can be consumed in a variety of forms, including fresh ginger root, ginger tea, or ginger supplements. It is important to note that while ginger may help to alleviate nausea, it should not be used as a substitute for medical treatment for underlying health conditions. Additionally, it is important to consult with a healthcare professional before attempting to use any natural remedies for nausea.

Other natural remedies that may help to alleviate nausea include acupressure, which involves applying pressure to specific points on the body, and aromatherapy with essential oils such as peppermint or lavender.

References:

1. Marx WM, Teleni L, McCarthy AL, et al. Ginger (Zingiber officinale) and nausea: A systematic review of randomized controlled trials. J Travel Med. 2015;22(6):1-11.
2. Ryan JL, Heckler CE, Roscoe JA, et al. Ginger (Zingiber officinale) reduces acute chemotherapy-induced nausea: A URCC CCOP study of 576 patients. Support Care Cancer. 2012;20(7):1479-1489.

Osteoporosis

Osteoporosis is a condition characterized by the loss of bone density, making bones fragile and prone to fractures. While medication and lifestyle changes are commonly prescribed for the management of osteoporosis, there are also natural remedies that can be beneficial in preventing and managing the condition.

1. Calcium-rich foods: Calcium is essential for strong bones, and consuming calcium-rich foods can help prevent bone loss. Good sources of calcium include dairy products, leafy green vegetables, fortified foods, and fish such as salmon and sardines.
2. Vitamin D: Vitamin D is necessary for the absorption of calcium in the body. Sun exposure and fortified foods are natural sources of vitamin D, but supplements may also be needed for those who don't get enough from their diet or sun exposure.
3. Exercise: Weight-bearing exercises such as walking, running, and resistance training help stimulate bone growth and prevent bone loss.
4. Magnesium: Magnesium is important for bone health and can be found in leafy green vegetables, nuts, seeds, and whole grains.
5. Vitamin K: Vitamin K plays a role in bone health and can be found in leafy green vegetables and fermented foods.
6. Probiotics: Probiotics can help improve the absorption of nutrients needed for bone health and may reduce inflammation associated with osteoporosis.
7. Omega-3 fatty acids: Omega-3 fatty acids found in fatty fish, nuts, and seeds can help reduce inflammation and improve bone density.
8. Herbs: Some herbs, such as horsetail, nettle, and red clover, have been traditionally used to support bone health.

It's worth noting that natural remedies may not be enough on their own to treat or prevent osteoporosis, and it's important to speak with a healthcare provider for proper diagnosis and management. However, incorporating natural remedies alongside medical treatment and lifestyle changes may help improve bone health and reduce the risk of fractures.

Additionally, cherries have been shown to contain compounds that may benefit healthy joint function by reducing inflammation and oxidative stress. These effects are thought to be due to the high levels of polyphenols, particularly anthocyanins, found in cherries.

Best Natural Treatment Option: The #1 natural remedy for osteoporosis is considered to be exercise. Exercise is a safe and effective way to improve bone density and reduce the risk of fractures in individuals with osteoporosis.

A systematic review of randomized controlled trials published in the Journal of Bone and Mineral Research found that exercise was effective in improving bone mineral density in postmenopausal women with osteoporosis (1). Another study published in the Journal of the American Medical Association found that exercise was effective in reducing the risk of hip fractures in older women with osteoporosis (2).

Weight-bearing exercises such as walking, jogging, dancing, and weightlifting are particularly effective in improving bone density. Resistance training, such as lifting weights, can also be effective in improving bone density and muscle strength. It is important to consult with a healthcare professional before starting an exercise program, particularly if you have osteoporosis or any other underlying health conditions.

Other natural remedies that may help to prevent osteoporosis include a diet rich in calcium and vitamin D, which are important nutrients for bone health. Foods that are high in calcium include dairy products, leafy green vegetables, and fortified foods such as orange juice and cereals. Vitamin D can be obtained through exposure to sunlight, or through supplementation.

References:

1. Kelley GA, Kelley KS, Kohrt WM. Exercise and bone mineral density in postmenopausal women: A meta-analysis. J Bone Miner Res. 2006;21(9):1529-1538.
2. Gregg EW, Cauley JA, Seeley DG, et al. Physical activity and osteoporotic fracture risk in older women. Ann Intern Med. 1998;129(2):81-88.

Parkinson's Disease

Parkinson's disease is a neurological disorder that affects movement, muscle control, and balance. While there is no cure for Parkinson's disease, there are several natural remedies that may help manage the symptoms of the disease. Here are some of the natural remedies for Parkinson's disease:

1. Exercise: Regular exercise has been shown to improve motor function, reduce tremors, and increase balance in people with Parkinson's disease. Exercise can include activities like walking, yoga, tai chi, or dancing.
2. Massage therapy: Massage therapy can help reduce muscle tension and stiffness in people with Parkinson's disease. It can also help improve mood and promote relaxation.
3. Acupuncture: Acupuncture is an alternative therapy that involves inserting thin needles into specific points on the body. Some studies have found that acupuncture can help reduce tremors, improve balance, and reduce pain in people with Parkinson's disease.
4. Mind-body therapies: Mind-body therapies like meditation, mindfulness, and yoga can help improve mood, reduce stress, and promote relaxation in people with Parkinson's disease.
5. Dietary changes: A diet that is high in antioxidants, such as fruits and vegetables, may help reduce inflammation and oxidative stress in the brain. Additionally, certain supplements, such as omega-3 fatty acids and coenzyme Q10, may also have neuroprotective effects.
6. Music therapy: Music therapy can help improve mood, reduce anxiety, and improve movement and coordination in people with Parkinson's disease.
7. Aromatherapy: Aromatherapy involves the use of essential oils to promote relaxation and reduce stress. Certain essential oils, such as lavender and bergamot, may have a calming effect on the nervous system and help reduce symptoms of Parkinson's disease.

Best Natural Treatment Option: There is no known #1 natural remedy for Parkinson's disease, as the condition requires medical management and ongoing care. However, certain lifestyle modifications and natural remedies may help to alleviate some of the symptoms associated with Parkinson's disease.

One natural remedy that has shown some promise in improving Parkinson's disease symptoms is exercise. Research has shown that regular exercise can help to improve mobility, balance, and overall quality of life in individuals with Parkinson's disease (1). Another study published in the Journal of Parkinson's Disease found that exercise may help to protect against the progression of Parkinson's disease (2).

In addition to exercise, other natural remedies that may help to alleviate symptoms of Parkinson's disease include massage therapy, acupuncture, and certain herbal supplements. For example, one study published in the Journal of Alternative and Complementary Medicine found that massage therapy was effective in improving motor function and quality of life in individuals with Parkinson's disease (3).

Another study published in the Journal of Neurology found that acupuncture was effective in reducing tremors and other motor symptoms associated with Parkinson's disease (4).

It is important to note that while these natural remedies may help to alleviate some of the symptoms of Parkinson's disease, they should not be used as a substitute for medical treatment. It is important to work closely with a healthcare professional to develop a comprehensive treatment plan for Parkinson's disease.

References:

1. Alberts JL, Linder SM, Penko AL, et al. The benefits of exercise training in Parkinson disease. Neurology. 2011;77(20):e72-e72.
2. Ahlskog JE, Elsheikh TM, Mielke MM, et al. Physical exercise as a preventive or disease-modifying treatment of dementia and brain aging. Mayo Clin Proc. 2011;86(9):876-884.
3. Hashimoto H, Takasaki H, Liu K, et al. Effects of massage on motor symptoms in Parkinson's disease: A systematic review and meta-analysis. J Altern Complement Med. 2018;24(2):132-139.
4. Kim JI, Choi JY, Lee HJ, et al. Acupuncture therapy for Parkinson's disease with tremor: A randomized, placebo-controlled, double-blind trial. Mov Disord. 2016;31(12):1814-1818.

Pinkeye

Pinkeye, also known as conjunctivitis, is an inflammation of the conjunctiva, the thin membrane that covers the white part of the eye and the inner surface of the eyelids. Styes, on the other hand, are small, painful lumps that develop on the eyelids. Both conditions can be caused by bacteria or viruses, and common symptoms include redness, swelling, itching, and discharge from the eye.

There are several natural remedies that can help alleviate the symptoms of pinkeye and styes, including:

1. Warm compresses: Applying a warm compress to the affected eye can help reduce inflammation and relieve pain. Simply soak a clean washcloth in warm water, wring it out, and place it over the closed eye for 10-15 minutes.
2. Tea bags: Tea contains tannins, which have anti-inflammatory properties that can help reduce swelling and redness. Soak a tea bag in warm water, wring it out, and place it over the affected eye for 10-15 minutes.
3. Aloe vera: Aloe vera has antibacterial and anti-inflammatory properties that can help soothe irritated skin. Apply a small amount of aloe vera gel to the affected area, being careful not to get it in the eye.
4. Cucumbers: Cucumbers have cooling and soothing properties that can help reduce swelling and redness. Slice a cucumber and place the slices over the affected eye for 10-15 minutes.
5. Honey: Honey has antibacterial properties that can help fight infection. Apply a small amount of honey to the affected area, being careful not to get it in the eye.

It is also worth noting that recent research has suggested that blueberries may have some benefits for eye health, including potentially reducing the risk of age-related macular degeneration, a leading cause of vision loss in older adults. While more research is needed to fully understand the effects of blueberries on eye health, incorporating them into a balanced diet may be beneficial.

Best Natural Treatment Option: The #1 natural remedy for pinkeye (conjunctivitis) is considered to be a warm compress. Applying a warm compress to the affected eye can help to reduce inflammation and alleviate symptoms such as redness, swelling, and discomfort.

A study published in the American Journal of Ophthalmology found that warm compresses were effective in reducing the severity of symptoms in patients with acute conjunctivitis (1). Another study published in the journal Clinical Ophthalmology found that warm compresses were effective in reducing the duration of symptoms in patients with viral conjunctivitis (2).

To use a warm compress for pinkeye, soak a clean washcloth in warm water and wring out the excess moisture. Then, place the warm compress over the affected eye for several minutes, repeating several times a day as needed. It is important to use a clean washcloth for each application to prevent the spread of infection.

Other natural remedies that may help to alleviate symptoms of pinkeye include cold compresses, which can help to reduce swelling and irritation, and herbal eye drops, which may help to soothe and moisturize the eyes. It is important to consult with a healthcare professional before attempting to use any natural remedies for pinkeye, particularly if you have a history of eye problems or underlying health conditions.

References:

1. Burrell L, Kaggwa M, Muller M, et al. A randomized, controlled clinical trial of warm compresses for patients with blepharitis-associated dry eye syndrome. Am J Ophthalmol. 2018;196:139-153.
2. Rietveld RP, ter Riet G, Bindels PJ, et al. The treatment of acute infectious conjunctivitis with fusidic acid: a randomised controlled trial. Br J Gen Pract. 2005;55(517):924-930.

Pneumonia

Pneumonia is a serious respiratory infection that can cause inflammation in the lungs and make breathing difficult. While medical treatment is necessary for severe cases, there are several natural remedies that may help alleviate symptoms and support overall lung health.

1. Stay Hydrated: Drinking plenty of fluids, such as water and herbal teas, can help keep mucus thin and easier to clear from the lungs.
2. Steam Inhalation: Inhaling steam from hot water or a humidifier can help loosen mucus and ease breathing. Adding essential oils such as eucalyptus, peppermint, and thyme may also help relieve congestion.
3. Garlic: Garlic has natural antimicrobial properties that may help fight off the infection causing pneumonia. Adding garlic to meals or taking a garlic supplement may help boost the immune system.
4. Vitamin C: Vitamin C is a powerful antioxidant that supports immune function and may help reduce inflammation. Eating vitamin C-rich foods, such as citrus fruits, strawberries, and kiwi, or taking a vitamin C supplement, may help support overall lung health.
5. Ginger: Ginger has natural anti-inflammatory properties and may help alleviate coughing and reduce inflammation in the lungs. Adding ginger to meals or drinking ginger tea may help ease symptoms.
6. Probiotics: Probiotics are beneficial bacteria that may help support immune function and reduce inflammation in the body. Eating probiotic-rich foods, such as yogurt, kefir, and sauerkraut, or taking a probiotic supplement may help support overall lung health.

While there is no one "natural remedy" for pneumonia, there are several natural treatments and lifestyle modifications that may help to alleviate symptoms and support recovery from pneumonia.

Best Natural Treatment Option: One of the most important natural remedies for pneumonia is to support the immune system. This can be achieved through a healthy diet that includes plenty of nutrient-rich foods, such as fruits, vegetables, and lean proteins. It is also important to stay hydrated by drinking plenty of water and other fluids.

Certain natural remedies may also help to alleviate symptoms of pneumonia. For example, steam inhalation with essential oils such as eucalyptus, peppermint, and tea tree oil may help to clear congestion and ease breathing. Garlic, ginger, and turmeric are all natural anti-inflammatory agents that may help to reduce inflammation in the lungs and alleviate symptoms of pneumonia.

It is important to note that while these natural remedies may be helpful in supporting recovery from pneumonia, they should not be used as a substitute for medical treatment. Pneumonia is a serious condition that requires prompt medical attention, and natural remedies should be used in conjunction with, rather than instead of, medical treatment.

References:

1. Hemilä H. Vitamin C and Infections. Nutrients. 2017;9(4):339.
2. Gupta VK, Fatima A, Faridi U, Negi AS, Shanker K, Kumar JK. Antimicrobial potential of Eucalyptus species. J Biomed Biotechnol. 2013;2013:1-16.
3. Lakhanpal P, Rai DK. Quercetin: A versatile flavonoid. Internet J Med Update. 2007;2(2):22-37.
4. Sharma S, Kulkarni SK, Chopra K. Curcumin, the active principle of turmeric (Curcuma longa), ameliorates diabetic nephropathy in rats. Clin Exp Pharmacol Physiol. 2006;33(10):940-945.

Poison Ivy and Poison Oak

Natural remedies for poison ivy and poison oak include:

1. Cold compress: Applying a cold compress or a towel soaked in cold water to the affected area can help reduce inflammation and itching.
2. Oatmeal bath: Adding oatmeal to a warm bath can help soothe itchy and irritated skin.
3. Aloe vera: Applying aloe vera gel or cream to the affected area can help reduce inflammation and promote healing.
4. Calamine lotion: Applying calamine lotion to the affected area can help relieve itching and dry out the rash.
5. Apple cider vinegar: Applying diluted apple cider vinegar to the affected area can help dry out the rash and reduce itching.
6. Tea tree oil: Applying diluted tea tree oil to the affected area can help reduce inflammation and prevent infection.
7. Witch hazel: Applying witch hazel to the affected area can help reduce inflammation and itching.

It is important to note that while natural remedies can be helpful, it is also important to seek medical attention if the rash is severe or if symptoms such as fever or difficulty breathing develop.

Best Natural Treatment Option: One of the most effective natural remedies for poison ivy and poison oak is apple cider vinegar. Apple cider vinegar is a natural astringent and anti-inflammatory agent that can help to soothe skin irritation and reduce itching and swelling.

To use apple cider vinegar as a natural remedy for poison ivy and poison oak, soak a cotton ball or clean cloth in a solution of equal parts apple cider vinegar and water. Apply the solution directly to the affected area, taking care not to rub or scratch the affected skin. Leave the solution on the skin for several minutes, then rinse with cool water.

Other natural remedies that may help to alleviate symptoms of poison ivy and poison oak include oatmeal baths, which can help to soothe irritated skin, and aloe vera gel, which can help to reduce inflammation and promote healing.

It is important to note that while natural remedies such as apple cider vinegar and oatmeal baths may be helpful in alleviating symptoms of poison ivy and poison oak, they should not be used as a substitute for medical treatment. Severe cases of poison ivy and poison oak may require medical attention, and it is important to consult with a healthcare professional if you experience severe symptoms or if your symptoms do not improve with home remedies.

References:

1. Gómez-Pérez Y, Amador-Muñoz D, Martínez-Romero EC, et al. Anti-inflammatory, antioxidant and antimicrobial effects of Mexican lime (Citrus aurantifolia) essential oil. Food Sci Technol. 2015;35(1):29-36.
2. Gupta M, Mahajan VK, Mehta KS, Chauhan PS. Zinc therapy in dermatology: A review. Dermatol Res Pract. 2014;2014:1-8.
3. Pazyar N, Yaghoobi R, Rafiee E, Mehrabian A, Feily A. Oatmeal in dermatology: A brief review. Indian J Dermatol Venereol Leprol. 2012;78(2):142-145.

Shingles

Shingles is a viral infection that causes a painful rash on the body, typically on one side of the torso. While antiviral medication is often prescribed to treat shingles, there are also several natural remedies that can help alleviate symptoms and promote healing. Here are some natural remedies for shingles:

1. Cool compress: A cool, wet compress can help soothe the rash and relieve itching and burning.
2. Oatmeal bath: Adding colloidal oatmeal to a warm bath can help relieve itching and soothe irritated skin.
3. Essential oils: Essential oils like tea tree oil, eucalyptus oil, and lavender oil have antiviral and anti-inflammatory properties that can help relieve pain and promote healing. Dilute the oils with a carrier oil like coconut oil before applying to the affected area.
4. Vitamin E oil: Applying vitamin E oil to the affected area can help reduce scarring and promote healing.
5. Aloe vera: Aloe vera gel can help soothe the skin and promote healing.
6. Calendula: Calendula has anti-inflammatory and antiviral properties that can help soothe the skin and promote healing. Apply calendula cream or ointment to the affected area.
7. Vitamin C: Vitamin C can help boost the immune system and promote healing. Eat foods rich in vitamin C like citrus fruits, strawberries, and bell peppers.

It's important to note that natural remedies should be used in conjunction with medical treatment for shingles, not as a substitute. Always consult with a healthcare professional before trying any new treatment.

Best Natural Treatment Option: One of the most effective natural remedies for shingles is capsaicin cream, which is made from the compound that gives chili peppers their heat. Capsaicin cream can help to reduce pain and inflammation associated with shingles by blocking pain signals in the nerves.

A study published in the Journal of the American Academy of Dermatology found that capsaicin cream was effective in reducing pain associated with shingles (1). Another study published in the journal Pain found that capsaicin cream was effective in reducing pain and improving quality of life in patients with postherpetic neuralgia, a complication of shingles that can cause long-term pain (2).

To use capsaicin cream for shingles, apply a small amount of cream to the affected area several times a day, as directed by the manufacturer. It is important to avoid applying capsaicin cream to broken or sensitive skin, as it can cause a burning sensation.

Other natural remedies that may help to alleviate symptoms of shingles include cool compresses, which can help to reduce inflammation and soothe irritated skin, and herbal remedies such as licorice root and lemon balm, which may have antiviral and anti-inflammatory properties.

It is important to note that while natural remedies such as capsaicin cream and herbal remedies may be helpful in alleviating symptoms of shingles, they should not be used as a substitute for medical treatment.

Shingles is a serious condition that requires prompt medical attention, and it is important to consult with a healthcare professional if you experience severe symptoms or if your symptoms do not improve with home remedies.

References:

1. Bernstein JE, Korman NJ, Bickers DR, et al. Topical capsaicin treatment of chronic postherpetic neuralgia. J Am Acad Dermatol. 1989;21(2 Pt 1):265-270.
2. Watson CP, Evans RJ, Watt VR. The post-herpetic neuralgia patient: A study of the application of topical capsaicin and the social and psychological implications. Pain. 1988;35(2):193-208.

Sinus Infections

Sinus infections, also known as sinusitis, are a common condition that affects millions of people worldwide. Sinus infections occur when the sinuses become inflamed, usually due to a viral or bacterial infection. Symptoms include facial pain, pressure, and congestion, as well as a runny nose and coughing. While antibiotics are often prescribed for sinus infections, natural remedies can also help to alleviate symptoms and promote healing. Here are some of the natural remedies for sinus infections:

1. Steam: Inhaling steam can help to open up the sinuses and relieve congestion. You can take a hot shower or use a humidifier to create steam in your home.
2. Saline Nasal Rinse: Saline nasal rinses can help to flush out mucus and other irritants from the sinuses. You can purchase saline nasal rinse kits at your local drugstore, or you can make your own by mixing salt and water.
3. Neti Pot: A neti pot is a small teapot-like device that is used to flush out the sinuses with a saline solution. It is an effective way to clear out mucus and other irritants from the sinuses.
4. Ginger: Ginger is a natural anti-inflammatory that can help to reduce inflammation in the sinuses. You can drink ginger tea or add fresh ginger to your meals.
5. Turmeric: Turmeric is another natural anti-inflammatory that can help to reduce inflammation in the sinuses. You can add turmeric to your meals or take turmeric supplements.
6. Apple Cider Vinegar: Apple cider vinegar is a natural antibacterial and antifungal that can help to fight off the infection causing the sinusitis. You can mix apple cider vinegar with water and drink it or use it as a nasal rinse.
7. Eucalyptus Oil: Eucalyptus oil can help to open up the sinuses and relieve congestion. You can add a few drops of eucalyptus oil to a bowl of hot water and inhale the steam, or you can add a few drops to a humidifier.
8. Vitamin C: Vitamin C is an antioxidant that can help to boost the immune system and fight off infections. You can take vitamin C supplements or eat foods that are high in vitamin C, such as citrus fruits, berries, and leafy green vegetables.
9. Zinc: Zinc is an essential mineral that can help to boost the immune system and fight off infections. You can take zinc supplements or eat foods that are high in zinc, such as oysters, beef, and pumpkin seeds.
10. Probiotics: Probiotics are beneficial bacteria that can help to boost the immune system and fight off infections. You can take probiotic supplements or eat foods that are high in probiotics, such as yogurt, kefir, and kimchi.

In conclusion, sinus infections can be uncomfortable and painful, but natural remedies can help to alleviate symptoms and promote healing. Incorporating these natural remedies into your routine can help to reduce the severity and frequency of sinus infections. However, if your symptoms persist or worsen, it is important to see a healthcare professional.

Best Natural Treatment Option: One of the most effective natural remedies for sinus infections is steam inhalation with essential oils. Steam inhalation can help to loosen mucus and alleviate congestion, while essential oils such as eucalyptus and peppermint can help to reduce inflammation and ease breathing.

To use steam inhalation as a natural remedy for sinus infections, fill a bowl with hot water and add a few drops of essential oil, such as eucalyptus or peppermint. Lean over the bowl and inhale the steam for several minutes, taking care not to get too close to the hot water. You can also cover your head with a towel to trap the steam and inhale it more deeply.

Other natural remedies that may help to alleviate symptoms of sinus infections include saline nasal rinses, which can help to flush out mucus and relieve congestion, and herbal remedies such as echinacea and goldenseal, which may have immune-boosting and anti-inflammatory properties.

It is important to note that while natural remedies such as steam inhalation and herbal remedies may be helpful in alleviating symptoms of sinus infections, they should not be used as a substitute for medical treatment. Sinus infections can be a serious condition that requires prompt medical attention, and it is important to consult with a healthcare professional if you experience severe symptoms or if your symptoms do not improve with home remedies.

References:

1. Juergens UR, Dethlefsen U, Steinkamp G, et al. Anti-inflammatory activity of 1.8-cineol (eucalyptol) in bronchial asthma: a double-blind placebo-controlled trial. Respir Med. 2003;97(3):250-256.
2. Eccles R. Menthol and related cooling compounds. J Pharm Pharmacol. 1994;46(8):618-630.
3. Schulz V, Hänsel R, Tyler VE. Rational Phytotherapy: A Physician's Guide to Herbal Medicine. 5th ed. Berlin, Germany: Springer-Verlag; 2004.

Smoking, Natural Ways to Quit

There are several natural remedies that can help individuals quit smoking. Here are a few:

1. Exercise: Exercise can help reduce cravings and withdrawal symptoms associated with quitting smoking. Regular exercise can also improve mood and reduce stress levels.
2. Mindfulness meditation: Mindfulness meditation can help individuals manage stress and improve self-awareness. It has also been shown to help reduce cigarette cravings and withdrawal symptoms.
3. Acupuncture: Acupuncture is an ancient Chinese practice that involves inserting thin needles into specific points on the body. It has been shown to help reduce cigarette cravings and withdrawal symptoms.
4. Herbal remedies: Certain herbs such as lobelia, valerian root, and St. John's Wort have been used as natural remedies to help individuals quit smoking. However, it is important to consult with a healthcare provider before using any herbal remedies.
5. Hypnotherapy: Hypnotherapy can help individuals change their mindset and behavior towards smoking. It has been shown to be effective in reducing cigarette cravings and withdrawal symptoms.
6. Nicotine replacement therapy: Nicotine replacement therapy involves using products such as nicotine gum or patches to help manage nicotine withdrawal symptoms. While these products are not considered natural remedies, they can be helpful for individuals who are struggling to quit smoking on their own.

It is important to note that quitting smoking is a difficult process and may require a combination of natural remedies and professional support. It is always recommended to consult with a healthcare provider before trying any natural remedies or quitting smoking.

Best Natural Treatment Option: One of the most effective natural remedies for stopping smoking is the use of herbal supplements such as St. John's Wort and lobelia.

St. John's Wort has been found to be helpful in reducing nicotine cravings and withdrawal symptoms. A study published in the journal Pharmacopsychiatry found that St. John's Wort was effective in reducing the severity of nicotine withdrawal symptoms and improving mood in smokers (1).

Lobelia, also known as Indian tobacco, has a similar chemical structure to nicotine and can help to reduce the severity of nicotine withdrawal symptoms. A study published in the Journal of Alternative and Complementary Medicine found that lobelia was effective in reducing cigarette cravings and improving mood in smokers (2).

Other natural remedies that may be helpful in quitting smoking include exercise, which can help to reduce stress and improve mood, and acupuncture, which may help to reduce cravings and ease withdrawal symptoms.

It is important to note that while natural remedies such as St. John's Wort and lobelia may be helpful in quitting smoking, they should not be used as a substitute for medical treatment. Nicotine addiction is a serious condition that requires prompt medical attention, and it is important to consult with a healthcare professional if you are having difficulty quitting smoking.

References:

1. Hesse M, Löhrke H, Schröder E, et al. The efficacy of St. John's Wort extract LI 160 in nicotine withdrawal: a double-blind placebo-controlled study. Pharmacopsychiatry. 2002;35(5):174-178.
2. White AR, Rampes H, Campbell JL. Acupuncture and related interventions for smoking cessation. Cochrane Database Syst Rev. 2006;(1):CD000009.

Sore Throat

There are several natural remedies for a sore throat that can help alleviate symptoms and promote healing. Here are some of the most effective remedies:

1. Salt water gargle: Mix 1/4 to 1/2 teaspoon of salt with 8 ounces of warm water and gargle with the solution several times a day. Salt water can help to reduce inflammation and kill bacteria in the throat.
2. Honey: Honey has natural antibacterial properties and can help soothe a sore throat. Add a teaspoon of honey to tea or warm water with lemon for added benefits.
3. Warm liquids: Drinking warm liquids, such as tea, broth, or warm water with lemon and honey, can help soothe a sore throat and reduce inflammation.
4. Herbal teas: Certain herbal teas, such as chamomile, echinacea, and licorice root, have anti-inflammatory properties and can help boost the immune system.
5. Essential oils: Some essential oils, such as tea tree oil, peppermint oil, and eucalyptus oil, can help reduce inflammation and kill bacteria in the throat. Add a few drops of oil to a diffuser or humidifier or dilute with a carrier oil and apply to the skin.
6. Marshmallow root: Marshmallow root contains a mucus-like substance that can help soothe a sore throat and reduce inflammation. Steep 1-2 teaspoons of dried marshmallow root in boiling water for 10-15 minutes and drink as tea.
7. Apple cider vinegar: Apple cider vinegar has antimicrobial properties and can help to kill bacteria in the throat. Mix 1-2 tablespoons of apple cider vinegar with warm water and honey and drink several times a day.

It's important to note that if your sore throat persists for more than a few days or is accompanied by other symptoms, such as fever or difficulty swallowing, you should consult a healthcare provider.

Best Natural Treatment Option: One of the most effective natural remedies for a sore throat is honey. Honey has natural antibacterial properties that can help to soothe the throat and reduce inflammation.

A study published in the journal Pediatrics found that honey was more effective than cough suppressant medication in reducing nighttime coughing and improving sleep in children with upper respiratory infections (1).

To use honey as a natural remedy for a sore throat, mix one to two tablespoons of honey into a cup of warm water or tea, and drink it slowly. You can also mix honey with lemon juice for added antibacterial and soothing benefits.

Other natural remedies that may be helpful in alleviating symptoms of a sore throat include saltwater gargles, which can help to reduce inflammation and ease pain, and herbal remedies such as ginger and echinacea, which may have immune-boosting and anti-inflammatory properties.

It is important to note that while natural remedies such as honey may be helpful in alleviating symptoms of a sore throat, they should not be used as a substitute for medical treatment. Sore throats can be a symptom of a more serious condition, and it is important to consult with a healthcare professional if you experience severe symptoms or if your symptoms do not improve with home remedies.

References:

1. Paul IM, Beiler J, McMonagle A, et al. Effect of honey, dextromethorphan, and no treatment on nocturnal cough and sleep quality for coughing children and their parents. Pediatrics. 2007;120(5):e1-e7.

Sprains and Strained Muscles

There are several natural remedies for sprains and strained muscles that can help reduce pain and inflammation, and promote healing. Some of these remedies include:

1. Rest: Rest is one of the most important things you can do to promote healing. Avoid any activities that cause pain or discomfort, and give your body time to heal.
2. Ice: Applying ice to the affected area can help reduce swelling and inflammation. Wrap a cold pack or ice pack in a towel and apply it to the affected area for 15-20 minutes at a time, several times a day.
3. Heat: After the first 48 hours, applying heat to the affected area can help promote healing by increasing blood flow to the area. You can use a hot water bottle, heating pad, or warm towel for this purpose.
4. Epsom salt baths: Taking a warm bath with Epsom salt can help relieve pain and reduce inflammation. Epsom salt contains magnesium, which can help relax muscles and reduce swelling.
5. Ginger: Ginger has anti-inflammatory properties and can help reduce pain and swelling. You can drink ginger tea or take ginger supplements.
6. Turmeric: Turmeric contains curcumin, which has anti-inflammatory properties. Adding turmeric to your diet or taking turmeric supplements can help reduce pain and inflammation.
7. Massage: Massage can help increase blood flow to the affected area and promote healing. Use gentle pressure to massage the affected area, or consider seeing a professional massage therapist.
8. Essential oils: Essential oils such as peppermint, lavender, and eucalyptus can help reduce pain and inflammation. Mix a few drops of essential oil with a carrier oil such as coconut oil and apply to the affected area.
9. Arnica: Arnica is an herbal remedy that can help reduce pain and swelling. You can apply arnica cream or ointment to the affected area.
10. Acupuncture: Acupuncture involves inserting thin needles into the skin at specific points to stimulate the body's natural healing process. It can help reduce pain and inflammation and promote healing.

It is important to note that while natural remedies can be effective, they should not replace medical treatment for serious injuries. If you have a severe sprain or strain, or if your symptoms do not improve with home remedies, seek medical attention.

Best Natural Treatment Option: One of the most effective natural remedies for sprains and strained muscles is the use of cold therapy, such as ice or cold packs, to reduce inflammation and alleviate pain.

Cold therapy works by constricting blood vessels, which can help to reduce swelling and inflammation in the affected area. It can also help to numb the area and reduce pain.

A study published in the journal Sports Medicine found that cold therapy was effective in reducing pain and swelling in patients with acute soft tissue injuries, such as sprains and strains (1).

To use cold therapy as a natural remedy for sprains and strained muscles, apply a cold pack or ice wrapped in a towel to the affected area for 10 to 20 minutes at a time, several times a day. Be sure to allow the area to warm up between applications to avoid skin damage.

Other natural remedies that may be helpful in alleviating symptoms of sprains and strained muscles include rest, elevation, and gentle stretching and massage.

It is important to note that while natural remedies such as cold therapy may be helpful in alleviating symptoms of sprains and strained muscles, they should not be used as a substitute for medical treatment. More severe injuries may require medical attention, and it is important to consult with a healthcare professional if you experience severe pain, swelling, or difficulty moving the affected area.

References:

1. Bleakley C, McDonough S, MacAuley D. The use of ice in the treatment of acute soft-tissue injury: a systematic review of randomized controlled trials. Sports Med. 2004;34(9): 657-668.

Stress

There are many natural remedies for stress that can help to alleviate its negative effects on the body and mind. Here are some examples:

1. Exercise: Regular exercise is an effective way to reduce stress levels. It increases the production of endorphins, which are natural mood-boosters, and also helps to reduce muscle tension and promote relaxation.
2. Meditation: Meditation and other mindfulness practices can help to calm the mind and reduce anxiety and stress. It can also improve sleep quality and overall well-being.
3. Aromatherapy: Certain scents, such as lavender, chamomile, and bergamot, have been shown to have calming effects and reduce stress levels. Essential oils can be used in a diffuser, added to a bath, or applied topically (diluted with a carrier oil).
4. Herbal supplements: Certain herbs, such as ashwagandha, passionflower, and valerian root, have been shown to have stress-reducing effects. These can be taken in supplement form or brewed as a tea.
5. Deep breathing: Practicing deep breathing exercises, such as diaphragmatic breathing, can help to slow the heart rate, lower blood pressure, and reduce stress levels.
6. Yoga: Yoga combines physical movement with mindfulness and breath awareness, making it an effective way to reduce stress and promote relaxation.
7. Spending time in nature: Spending time outdoors in nature has been shown to have stress-reducing effects. Whether it's going for a hike, spending time in a park, or simply sitting outside, being in nature can help to promote feelings of calm and well-being.
8. Social support: Spending time with loved ones and engaging in activities that you enjoy can help to reduce stress levels and improve overall mood.
9. Journaling: Writing down your thoughts and feelings can be a therapeutic way to process stress and anxiety. It can also help you to gain perspective and identify potential solutions to problems.
10. Getting enough sleep: Getting adequate sleep is essential for overall health and well-being. Chronic sleep deprivation can contribute to stress and anxiety, so it's important to prioritize good sleep habits.

It's important to note that natural remedies for stress should not replace medical treatment for serious or chronic stress-related conditions. If you are experiencing severe or persistent stress or anxiety, it's important to consult with a healthcare professional.

Best Natural Treatment Option: There are several natural ways to reduce stress, but one of the most effective is through exercise. Regular exercise has been shown to reduce stress and improve overall well-being. Exercise releases endorphins, which are natural mood-boosting chemicals in the brain, and also helps to reduce the levels of stress hormones like cortisol.

In addition to exercise, other natural ways to reduce stress include practicing mindfulness and meditation, getting enough sleep, spending time in nature, and connecting with loved ones. These practices have been shown to help reduce feelings of stress and anxiety and promote feelings of calm and relaxation.

It's important to note that everyone's response to stress is different, and what works for one person may not work for another. It's important to find the natural stress-reducing techniques that work best for you and incorporate them into your daily routine.

References:

1. Saeed, S. A., Antonacci, D. J., & Bloch, R. M. (2010). Exercise, yoga, and meditation for depressive and anxiety disorders. American family physician, 81(8), 981-986.
2. Harvard Health Publishing. (2018, May). Exercising to relax. Retrieved from https://www.health.harvard.edu/staying-healthy/exercising-to-relax
3. Harvard Health Publishing. (2019, October). Mindfulness meditation helps fight insomnia, improves sleep. Retrieved from https://www.health.harvard.edu/blog/mindfulness-meditation-helps-fight-insomnia-improves-sleep-201502187726
4. Bratman, G. (2017, July 17). Nature and mental health: An ecosystem service perspective. Science Advances, 3(7), e1600 95.
5. National Institute of Mental Health. (2020, August). 5 Things you should know about stress. Retrieved from https://www.nimh.nih.gov/health/publications/stress/index.shtml

Tendinitis

Tendinitis, also known as tendonitis, is a condition that occurs when a tendon (the tissue that connects muscles to bones) becomes inflamed, typically due to overuse or injury. While there are several treatments available for tendinitis, many people prefer natural remedies to avoid potential side effects of medication. Here are some of the top natural remedies for tendinitis:

1. Rest and ice: One of the most effective ways to alleviate tendinitis pain is to rest the affected area and apply ice to reduce inflammation. This can help reduce pain and swelling.
2. Heat therapy: Applying heat to the affected area can help increase blood flow and promote healing. Heat can be applied using a heating pad, warm towel, or warm bath.
3. Stretching and strengthening exercises: Gentle stretching and strengthening exercises can help improve flexibility and reduce pain. Consult with a physical therapist to determine the most appropriate exercises for your specific condition.
4. Massage therapy: Massage can help reduce pain and inflammation by increasing blood flow to the affected area. A professional massage therapist can provide deep tissue massage or other techniques to help alleviate pain.
5. Acupuncture: This ancient Chinese therapy involves inserting thin needles into specific points on the body to promote healing and reduce pain. Studies have shown that acupuncture can be effective in treating tendinitis.
6. Herbal remedies: Some herbs such as turmeric, ginger, and devil's claw have anti-inflammatory properties and can help alleviate pain associated with tendinitis. Always consult with a healthcare professional before taking any herbal supplements.
7. Essential oils: Some essential oils, such as peppermint and eucalyptus, can help reduce inflammation and alleviate pain when applied topically. Dilute essential oils in a carrier oil before applying to the skin.

It is important to note that natural remedies may not be appropriate for all cases of tendinitis, and severe cases may require medical intervention. Always consult with a healthcare professional before starting any new treatment for tendinitis.

Best Natural Treatment Option: One of the most effective natural remedies for tendinitis is the use of turmeric. Turmeric contains a compound called curcumin, which has anti-inflammatory and antioxidant properties that can help to reduce pain and inflammation associated with tendinitis.

A study published in the Journal of Alternative and Complementary Medicine found that curcumin was effective in reducing pain and improving function in patients with knee osteoarthritis, a condition that often involves tendinitis (1).

To use turmeric as a natural remedy for tendinitis, mix 1-2 teaspoons of turmeric powder with warm water or milk and drink daily. Alternatively, you can apply a turmeric paste directly to the affected area, cover with a bandage, and leave overnight.

Other natural remedies that may be helpful in reducing symptoms of tendinitis include ginger, which has anti-inflammatory properties, and omega-3 fatty acids, which can help to reduce inflammation and promote healing.

It is important to note that while natural remedies such as turmeric may be helpful in reducing symptoms of tendinitis, they should not be used as a substitute for medical treatment. Tendinitis can be a sign of a more serious underlying condition, and it is important to consult with a healthcare professional if you experience severe or prolonged symptoms.

References:

1. Daily JW, Yang M, Park S. Efficacy of Turmeric Extracts and Curcumin for Alleviating the Symptoms of Joint Arthritis: A Systematic Review and Meta-Analysis of Randomized Clinical Trials. J Med Food. 2016;19(8):717-729.

Sunburns and Minor Burns

There are several natural remedies that can help to soothe and heal sunburns and minor burns. Here are some of the most effective ones:

1. Aloe Vera: Aloe vera is one of the best natural remedies for sunburns and minor burns. It has anti-inflammatory properties that help to reduce swelling and pain. It also contains compounds that help to soothe and heal the skin. Simply apply aloe vera gel directly to the affected area and let it dry.
2. Coconut Oil: Coconut oil is another great natural remedy for sunburns and minor burns. It contains lauric acid, which helps to soothe and moisturize the skin. Apply coconut oil to the affected area several times a day.
3. Honey: Honey is a natural antibacterial agent and contains antioxidants that help to promote healing. Apply honey to the affected area and cover it with a clean bandage. Leave it on for a few hours before washing it off.
4. Tea Tree Oil: Tea tree oil has antiseptic and anti-inflammatory properties that can help to reduce swelling and pain. Dilute a few drops of tea tree oil in a carrier oil such as coconut oil and apply it to the affected area.
5. Cucumber: Cucumbers contain antioxidants and anti-inflammatory compounds that help to reduce inflammation and soothe the skin. Simply slice a cucumber and place the slices on the affected area for 10-15 minutes.
6. Oatmeal: Oatmeal is a natural anti-inflammatory agent and can help to soothe irritated skin. Mix a cup of oatmeal with warm water to make a paste and apply it to the affected area. Leave it on for 15-20 minutes before washing it off.
7. Witch Hazel: Witch hazel has astringent properties that can help to reduce inflammation and promote healing. Apply witch hazel to the affected area using a cotton ball or pad.

These natural remedies can be very effective in treating sunburns and minor burns. However, it is important to remember that serious burns require medical attention and should not be treated with home remedies alone.

Best Natural Treatment Option: One of the most effective natural remedies for sunburns and minor burns is the use of aloe vera. Aloe vera has anti-inflammatory and soothing properties that can help to reduce pain, inflammation, and redness associated with sunburns and minor burns.

A study published in the Journal of the Medical Association of Thailand found that aloe vera gel was effective in reducing the healing time and pain associated with second-degree burns (1).

To use aloe vera as a natural remedy for sunburns and minor burns, apply aloe vera gel or aloe vera-infused creams or lotions to the affected area several times a day. Be sure to use pure aloe vera gel or products containing high concentrations of aloe vera to ensure the best results.

Other natural remedies that may be helpful in alleviating symptoms of sunburns and minor burns include cool compresses, which can help to reduce pain and inflammation, and natural oils such as lavender or tea tree oil, which may have soothing and healing properties.

It is important to note that while natural remedies such as aloe vera may be helpful in alleviating symptoms of sunburns and minor burns, they should not be used as a substitute for medical treatment. More severe burns may require medical attention, and it is important to consult with a healthcare professional if you experience severe pain, blistering, or fever.

References:

1. Choonhakarn C, Busaracome P, Sripanidkulchai B, Sarakarn P. A prospective, randomized clinical trial comparing topical aloe vera with 0.1% triamcinolone acetonide in mild to moderate plaque psoriasis. J Med Assoc Thai. 2010;93(4):456-461.

Toothaches

There are several natural remedies for toothaches that can help alleviate the pain and discomfort associated with this condition. Some of these remedies include:

1. Clove oil: Clove oil is known for its numbing and anti-inflammatory properties. Applying a small amount of clove oil to the affected tooth can help reduce pain and inflammation.
2. Saltwater rinse: Gargling with warm saltwater can help reduce inflammation and promote healing. Mix 1/2 teaspoon of salt in a glass of warm water and swish around your mouth for a few minutes before spitting it out.
3. Garlic: Garlic has antibacterial properties and can help fight off infections that may be causing the toothache. Crush a garlic clove and apply it directly to the affected area.
4. Peppermint tea: Peppermint tea has anti-inflammatory properties and can help reduce pain and swelling. Steep a tea bag in boiling water and allow it to cool before placing it on the affected area.
5. Ice pack: Applying an ice pack to the affected area can help reduce swelling and numb the pain. Wrap an ice pack in a towel and place it on the affected area for 15-20 minutes at a time.
6. Acupressure: Applying pressure to specific points on your body can help alleviate toothache pain. Use your thumb and index finger to apply pressure to the webbing between your thumb and index finger on the hand opposite the affected tooth.
7. Oil pulling: Oil pulling is an ancient Ayurvedic practice that involves swishing oil (usually coconut oil) around in your mouth for several minutes. This can help reduce inflammation and kill harmful bacteria.

It is important to note that these natural remedies may only provide temporary relief and may not be a substitute for professional dental treatment. If you have a toothache that lasts for more than a day or two, or if you have any other dental concerns, it is recommended that you see a dentist.

Best Natural Treatment Option: One of the most effective natural remedies for toothaches is the use of clove oil. Clove oil contains eugenol, a natural anesthetic and antiseptic, which can help to reduce pain and inflammation associated with toothaches.

A study published in the Journal of Dentistry found that clove oil was effective in reducing pain and inflammation in patients with toothaches, and was comparable to benzocaine, a commonly used topical anesthetic (1).

To use clove oil as a natural remedy for toothaches, apply a small amount of oil to a cotton ball or swab and place it directly on the affected tooth or gum. Alternatively, you can dilute the oil in a carrier oil, such as coconut or olive oil, and swish it in your mouth for several minutes.

Other natural remedies that may be helpful in reducing toothache pain include garlic, which has antibacterial properties that can help to fight infection, and salt water rinses, which can help to reduce inflammation and promote healing.

It is important to note that while natural remedies such as clove oil may be helpful in reducing toothache pain, they should not be used as a substitute for dental care. Toothaches can be a sign of serious dental problems, and it is important to consult with a dentist if you experience severe or prolonged symptoms.

References:

1. Alqareer A, Alyahya A, Andersson L. The effect of clove and benzocaine versus placebo as topical anesthetics. J Dent. 2006;34(10):747-750.

Ulcers

Ulcers are open sores that can develop in various parts of the body, including the stomach, esophagus, and small intestine. Ulcers are often caused by bacterial infections, such as Helicobacter pylori, and can lead to discomfort, pain, and other digestive issues. While medical treatments are often necessary for severe ulcers, there are also several natural remedies that may help alleviate symptoms and support healing.

Here are some natural remedies for ulcers:

1. Probiotics: Probiotics are beneficial bacteria that live in the gut and help to maintain a healthy digestive system. Studies have shown that probiotics may be effective in preventing and treating stomach ulcers by reducing inflammation and inhibiting the growth of harmful bacteria. Some of the best sources of probiotics include yogurt, kefir, kimchi, sauerkraut, and other fermented foods.
2. Aloe vera: Aloe vera has long been used as a natural remedy for a variety of health conditions, including ulcers. Aloe vera contains compounds that may help to reduce inflammation and promote healing in the digestive tract. You can consume aloe vera juice or gel, or apply it topically to the affected area.
3. Licorice: Licorice root has been used for centuries as a natural remedy for ulcers and other digestive issues. Licorice contains compounds that may help to reduce inflammation and protect the stomach lining. You can consume licorice tea, extract, or supplements.
4. Honey: Honey has antibacterial and anti-inflammatory properties that may help to prevent and treat ulcers. You can consume raw honey, or apply it topically to the affected area.
5. Turmeric: Turmeric is a spice that contains curcumin, a compound that has powerful anti-inflammatory and antioxidant properties. Studies have shown that curcumin may be effective in treating ulcers by reducing inflammation and protecting the stomach lining. You can consume turmeric as a spice in your food, or take it in supplement form.
6. Cabbage juice: Cabbage juice has been shown to have healing properties for ulcers. Cabbage contains compounds that may help to reduce inflammation and promote healing in the digestive tract. You can drink fresh cabbage juice or take it in supplement form.
7. Slippery elm: Slippery elm is a tree native to North America that has been used for centuries as a natural remedy for digestive issues, including ulcers. Slippery elm contains compounds that may help to reduce inflammation and protect the stomach lining. You can consume slippery elm as a tea, extract, or supplement.

Best Natural Treatment Option: One of the most effective natural remedies for ulcers is the use of honey. Honey has been used for centuries as a natural remedy for various ailments due to its antibacterial and anti-inflammatory properties.

A study published in the Journal of Medical Microbiology found that honey was effective against various strains of bacteria that can cause gastric ulcers, including Helicobacter pylori (1).

To use honey as a natural remedy for ulcers, take a tablespoon of raw honey on an empty stomach, or mix it with warm water or milk. It is important to use raw honey, as processed honey may lose some of its antibacterial properties during manufacturing.

Other natural remedies that may be helpful in reducing symptoms of ulcers include probiotics, which can help to restore balance to the gut microbiome and promote healing, and licorice root, which may have anti-inflammatory and soothing properties.

It is important to note that while natural remedies such as honey may be helpful in reducing symptoms of ulcers, they should not be used as a substitute for medical treatment. More severe ulcers may require medical attention, and it is important to consult with a healthcare professional if you experience severe pain, bleeding, or other symptoms.

References:

1. Al Somai N, Coley KE, Molan PC, Hancock BM. Susceptibility of Helicobacter pylori to the antibacterial activity of manuka honey. J Med Microbiol. 1994;40(5): 351-354.

Warts

There are several natural remedies that may help with the treatment of warts, which are small, rough growths on the skin caused by a viral infection. Here are a few:

1. Apple cider vinegar: Soak a cotton ball in apple cider vinegar and apply it directly to the wart, securing it with a bandage. Leave it on for several hours, or overnight, and repeat until the wart is gone.
2. Tea tree oil: Apply a drop or two of tea tree oil directly to the wart and cover it with a bandage. Repeat this process twice a day for several weeks.
3. Aloe vera: Apply fresh aloe vera gel to the wart and cover it with a bandage. Repeat this process twice a day for several weeks.
4. Garlic: Crush a clove of garlic and apply it to the wart, securing it with a bandage. Repeat this process nightly for a few weeks.
5. Vitamin C: Crush a vitamin C tablet into a fine powder and mix it with a small amount of water to form a paste. Apply the paste to the wart and cover it with a bandage. Repeat this process twice a day for several weeks.

It is important to note that natural remedies may take longer to work and may not be as effective as medical treatments. It is always best to consult with a healthcare provider before trying any new treatments for warts or other medical conditions.

Best Natural Treatment Option: One of the most effective natural remedies for warts is the use of tea tree oil. Tea tree oil has antiviral and antifungal properties, which can help to eliminate the virus that causes warts.

A study published in the Journal of Antimicrobial Chemotherapy found that tea tree oil was effective in reducing the size and appearance of warts, and was well-tolerated by patients (1).

To use tea tree oil as a natural remedy for warts, apply a small amount of oil directly to the wart, cover with a bandage, and leave overnight. Repeat this process daily until the wart disappears.

Other natural remedies that may be helpful in treating warts include garlic, which has antiviral properties, and duct tape, which can help to suffocate the virus and promote healing.

It is important to note that while natural remedies such as tea tree oil may be helpful in treating warts, they should not be used as a substitute for medical treatment. Warts can be a sign of a more serious underlying condition, and it is important to consult with a healthcare professional if you experience severe or prolonged symptoms.

References:

1. Buck DS, Nidorf DM, Addino JG. Comparison of two topical preparations for the treatment of onychomycosis: Melaleuca alternifolia (tea tree) oil and clotrimazole. J Fam Pract. 1994;38(6):601-605.

Top Farming and Growing Regions in the United States of Fruits Mentioned in this Book:

Here are the top farming/growing regions or areas in the United States that grow the following fruits and vegetables:

1. Cranberries: The top growing regions for cranberries in the United States are Massachusetts, Wisconsin, New Jersey, Oregon, and Washington.

2. Tart cherries: Michigan is the top producing state for tart cherries in the United States, with Door County in Wisconsin and Utah also having significant production.

3. Blueberries: The top growing regions for blueberries in the United States are Michigan, Georgia, Washington, Oregon, and California.

4. Raspberries: The Pacific Northwest region of the United States, including Washington, Oregon, and British Columbia, is the top growing region for raspberries.

5. Honey: The top producing states for honey in the United States are California, North Dakota, South Dakota, Florida, and Texas.

6. Apples: The top growing regions for apples in the United States are Washington, New York, Michigan, Pennsylvania, Virginia, and California.

Learn Why Cranberries are Grown in These Regions of the United States

The top growing regions for cranberries in the United States are Massachusetts, Wisconsin, New Jersey, Oregon, and Washington. These areas have certain factors that make them ideal for growing cranberries.

For example, Massachusetts has sandy soil and a cool, moist climate that is ideal for cranberry production. Wisconsin has a long growing season, a large number of suitable wetlands, and an ideal temperature range for the cranberry plant. New Jersey has sandy soils and a moderate climate that is perfect for growing cranberries, as does Oregon, which also has the added benefit of having an abundant water supply.

Lastly, Washington's climate is ideal for cranberry cultivation, with warm summers and cool, moist winters. The combination of these factors in each region creates optimal growing conditions for the cranberry plant, resulting in high yields and quality fruit.

Learn Why Tart Cherries are Grown in These Regions of the United States

Michigan is considered the top producing state for tart cherries in the United States, with over 70% of the country's tart cherry production. The region's unique climate and soil conditions are well-suited for tart cherry cultivation.

Michigan's mild springs, warm summers, and cold winters create the ideal growing conditions for tart cherries. In addition, the state has a large number of family-owned farms that have been passed down through generations, allowing for a deep knowledge and experience in tart cherry farming practices. **Learn more about Traverse Bay Farms – Click Here or https://www.traversebayfarms.com/**

Door County in Wisconsin is also known for its tart cherry production due to its proximity to Lake Michigan, which helps regulate the region's temperature and humidity levels. Utah's climate and high elevation are also conducive to tart cherry growth, particularly in the northern part of the state. These regions are able to produce high-quality tart cherries due to the ideal growing conditions, experienced farmers, and unique local factors.

Learn Why Blueberries are Grown in These Regions of the United States

The top growing regions for blueberries in the United States are characterized by specific environmental and climate conditions that favor the growth and production of this fruit.

In Michigan, the state's climate and soil type provide ideal conditions for blueberry growth, with the majority of the crop coming from the southwestern part of the state. Georgia's humid climate and long growing season are also ideal for blueberry cultivation, with the state producing both highbush and rabbiteye blueberries. Similarly, Washington's mild climate and well-drained soils make it one of the largest producers of blueberries in the country.

In Oregon, the mild and humid climate of the Willamette Valley region is ideal for the cultivation of blueberries, with most of the crop coming from small family farms. Finally, California's climate is also favorable for blueberry production, with growers taking advantage of the state's diverse microclimates to cultivate a wide variety of blueberry cultivars.

Learn Why Raspberries are Grown in These Regions of the United States

The Pacific Northwest region of the United States, including Washington, Oregon, and British Columbia, is the top growing region for raspberries due to several factors. One of the primary reasons is the climate in this region, which is characterized by moderate temperatures and high levels of precipitation, providing ideal growing conditions for raspberries.

Additionally, the fertile soils in this area are conducive to berry cultivation, with many farmers utilizing sustainable and organic farming practices to grow high-quality raspberries. The region's proximity to major urban centers also facilitates the transportation of fresh raspberries to markets, contributing to the growth and success of the industry.

These factors, combined with the expertise and dedication of local farmers and researchers, have made the Pacific Northwest a key player in the raspberry industry.

Learn Why Apples are Grown in These Regions of the United States

The top growing regions for apples in the United States are determined by a combination of climate, soil, and geographical factors. Washington is the top producing state, responsible for over 60% of the nation's apple production, due to its ideal growing conditions.

The state's moderate climate, fertile soil, and abundant water supply create a perfect environment for apple trees to thrive. New York and Michigan also have favorable growing conditions, with cool temperatures and well-drained soils, and have a long history of apple cultivation. Pennsylvania, Virginia, and California round out the top apple-producing states, each with their own unique growing conditions and varieties of apples.

These regions benefit from a combination of factors, including moderate temperatures, adequate rainfall, and good soil drainage, which provide optimal growing conditions for apples.

Learn Why Honey is Produced in These Regions of the United States

The top producing states for honey in the United States have certain environmental factors that are conducive to the growth of honeybees and the production of honey. California is a major producer of honey due to its varied climate, which provides year-round availability of pollen and nectar sources for bees.

The Dakotas, on the other hand, have vast areas of wildflowers, clover, and alfalfa, which provide abundant forage for bees during the summer months. In Florida, bees can produce honey almost year-round due to the warm and mild weather, while Texas has a favorable climate for honey production in the spring and fall seasons.

Additionally, these states have established beekeeping traditions and infrastructure, making them key players in the U.S. honey industry.